Praise for *Recovering You*

"Steven Washington shows us how recovery is a journey of rediscovery that can lead us back to our most authentic selves. I highly recommend *Recovering You* to anyone who is struggling with their identity for any reason."

— **Kristine Carlson**, coauthor of the
Don't Sweat the Small Stuff books

"Steven Washington shines as brightly as his words in this memoir turned road map to peace and acceptance. *Recovering You* is that light you've been asking for, and Steven is that friend you've prayed for. Your recovery has already begun."

— **Mike Dooley**, *New York Times* bestselling author of
Infinite Possibilities and *Notes from the Universe*

"A brilliant fusion of Steven Washington's understanding of the recovery road, his beautiful memoir-style writing, and a masterful guide to self-care and qigong all in one, this book is a gift for any reader looking to thrive. Having lived with Steven for seven years, I can attest that his daily devotion to self-care (in all its forms) is unwavering and has radically changed his life. May *Recovering You* do the same for you."

— **Lee Harris**, author of *Energy Speaks*
and the Conversations with the Z's series

"In *Recovering You*, Steven Washington states that he intends it 'to function as only a small piece of anyone's larger journey of recovery.' I beg to differ. In sharing such a comprehensive and invaluable range of tools, practices, insights, exercises, and experiences, he's created the definitive recovery bible for anyone at any — indeed, every — stage of their recovery journey."

— **Sandie Sedgbeer**, author, host of the *What is Going Om* radio
show, and founder of the No BS Spiritual Book Club

"This wise and thoughtful book offers a practical pathway to healing in understandable, down-to-earth language. Steven Washington's willingness to share his own dark nights, deep in addiction, negativity, and fear, makes him approachable and believable. Are you ready to explore your own self-worth and begin choosing your own happiness? *Recovering You* is chock-full of tools to support your journey. It's an open invitation to meet yourself where you are in this moment and move toward your highest potential. Isn't it time to choose you?"

— **Jane Beach**, author of *Freedom: Free to Be Me*

"*Recovering You* is a truly special journey. Steven Washington combines his calm and compassionate narrative with personal stories, wonderful and practical guidance, and the seamless weaving of considerations from friends in recovery as well. It feels more like stepping onto a path of clarity rather than reading a book. This is not a book to rush through, but one to savor and take time with. Many books focus only on logical or mental aspects, but *Recovering You* also delves into emotional, spiritual, and physical healing. Many sections caused me to reflect on aspects of my own life that I can't ever remember seeing in this way before. Steven's humble and honest voice allows you to drop your guard and feel at peace with exactly where you are. I highly recommend this book."

— **Doe Zantamata**, author of the Happiness in Your Life series

"*Recovering You* is a powerful contribution to the healing arts community. It is a thoughtfully written compilation of innovative ideas for self-care and wholistic healing. Steven Washington's expertise and finesse in teaching qigong can have a profoundly positive impact on your nervous system and sense of self. The way Steven uses the ancient practice of qigong with Western research and his own expertise is truly brilliant. Highly recommended for those reclaiming power within themselves."

— **Lee Holden**, TV personality, producer, author, and qigong master teacher

"*Recovering You* offers an understanding from personal experience of the journey from addiction to the gift of lasting recovery and ultimate freedom. Steven Washington is a beautiful soul, and his spirit and passion come through in his writing. Offering a set of tools and techniques, this is a must-read for anyone struggling with addiction and attempting to live in recovery with a sense of well-being, happiness, joy, and freedom."

— **Anita Moorjani**,
New York Times bestselling author of *Dying to Be Me*

"Compassionate, clear, intimate, and insightful, this book truly encompasses a full spectrum of wisdom and practical guidance for anyone in recovery who is looking for something more, something a little deeper, something that will enhance and add to the traditional approach to healing addiction. It addresses not just the mind, heart, and spirit but also the body. Each chapter takes you into one aspect of the sobriety journey and then invites you to embody the energy through specific movements. Those exercises provide the missing link, the key to experiencing a genuine but gentle breakthrough and allowing the healing, epiphanies, and intuitive knowing to be integrated and become undeniable. You find yourself on a bridge toward knowing that hope is tangible and real and that new beginnings open up to extraordinary potential and possibility as faith and forgiveness lead the way to freedom. As a person with long-term sobriety, I have read many books on recovery over the years, but I can honestly say this book stands out as my ultimate favorite, a much-needed guide for our modern times. Highly recommended."

— **Colette Baron-Reid**, author, educator, speaker, and artist

"As a person who has never had to face the journey of overcoming an addiction, I didn't think this would be a book for me. But from the start, I knew it would be a powerful book to help me release limiting habits. Steven Washington makes it clear that it is for anyone who wants to move past unproductive behaviors that keep them stuck and not able to move forward. He offers you tools and holds your hand through his writing so you can discover your courage and step into living a life of joy. You might not even remember what it feels like to be empowered, strong, free, and have a love for life, or yourself. But Steven can take you to that reality of awe and wonder and, as he says, to find your 'sober groove.' It is truly possible to be triumphant, and through *Recovering You*, Steven is the ideal guide to lead you to that triumph!"

— **Dondi Dahlin**, bestselling author of
The Five Elements

RECOVERING
YOU

Soul Care
and Mindful Movement
for Overcoming Addiction

STEVEN
WASHINGTON

New World Library
Novato, California

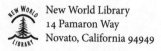

New World Library
14 Pamaron Way
Novato, California 94949

Text design by Tona Pearce Myers
Illustrations by Erin Posanti

Library of Congress Cataloging-in-Publication Data

Names: Washington, Steven Evan, author.
Title: Recovering you : soul care and mindful movement for overcoming
    addiction / Steven Washington.
Description: Novato, California : New World Library, [2022] | Includes
    bibliographical references. | Summary: "A holistic approach to overcoming
    addictive behavior using meditation, movement, and motivational
    techniques"-- Provided by publisher.
Identifiers: LCCN 2022022497 (print) | LCCN 2022022498 (ebook) |
    ISBN 9781608687954 (paperback) | ISBN 9781608687961 (ebook)
Subjects: LCSH: Addicts--Rehabilitation. | Meditation--Therapeutic use. | Movement therapy. | Spiritual life.
Classification: LCC HV4998 .W37 2022 (print) | LCC HV4998 (ebook) | DDC
    616.86/06--dc23/eng/20220801
LC record available at https://lccn.loc.gov/2022022497
LC ebook record available at https://lccn.loc.gov/2022022498

First printing, November 2022
ISBN 978-1-60868-795-4
Ebook ISBN 978-1-60868-796-1
Printed in Canada on 100% postconsumer-waste recycled paper

New World Library is proud to be a Gold Certified Environmentally Responsible Publisher. Publisher certification awarded by Green Press Initiative.

10   9   8   7   6   5   4   3   2   1

This book is dedicated to anyone anywhere who is in the struggle to find their way to freedom. May you find that which you seek.

CONTENTS

INTRODUCTION

Welcome. I have written this book for anyone who wants to be free of addictions, addictive behaviors, or negative habits of any kind. My goal is to provide a holistic pathway to an easier, kinder way of life that helps you move past the constraints that addictions and negative habits can create. This pathway is designed to meet you wherever you are on your trek toward autonomy and to help you cultivate the freedom to become the person you want to be. In the pages that follow, I provide a variety of tools, practices, movement techniques, reflections, personal examples, and healing conversations to help you feel more intimately connected to yourself and your life. I'm grateful to have this opportunity to connect with you through this book and to share my experience, strength, and hope in ways that, ideally, will be transformative for you.

A wise person once told me that we can't keep what we have unless we share it with others. I've taken that to heart, and for the past nineteen years, I've helped people through the important process of entering addiction recovery and tried to guide them through the turbulent and triumphant experiences that we in recovery can have. In more recent years, I've also been teaching movement and other wellness practices and incorporating them into addiction recovery. Through my studies and experiences, I have learned how powerful movement is for healing. I started my movement journey with dance, and along the way I have incorporated other movement-based practices like Pilates, qigong, and massage — all of which have helped me throughout my recovery.

Chinese medicine teaches that we hold emotions in the tissues of the body, and yet energy within the body and in nature is designed to flow freely. When it doesn't flow, it causes stagnation and many forms of disease. This stagnation negatively affects the body, mind, and spirit. However, mindful movement along with focused deep breathing helps eliminate stagnation and release long-held emotions and tension. If you adopt no other practices from this book, I hope you will make mindful movement a daily part of your recovery journey.

I have had the privilege of teaching this book's recovery techniques to people around the world, both online and at live events. Most people that I have worked with would classify themselves as sensitives, people who feel very deeply. They study with me to develop healthy ways to navigate their world and to manage their sensitivities to the energies of the people, places, and things in their lives. In my observations of myself and others in recovery over the years, I've seen a correlation between addiction and high sensitivity. Whether I'm leading groups or working with people in private, one-on-one sessions, I'm always moved by our shared journey. For all our kaleidoscopic differences, we are also so much alike.

The Connection between Freedom and Recovery

For the most part, everyone needs, wants, and longs for the same things. When I ask people what they really want, I often hear some version of "I want to be free…":

> "I want to be free from my addiction to overworking and overeating."
> "I want to be free from my addiction to drugs and alcohol."
> "I want to be free from stress and overwhelm."
> "I want to be free from anxiety, self-doubt, and fear."
> "I want to be free from depression and shame."
> "I want to be free from worrying about what others think of me."
> "I want to be free from physical pain."
> "I want to be free from the patterns of the past."
> "I want to be free from this sadness that never seems to go away."

I think that far too often many people feel trapped. Trapped by the demands of the present. Trapped by events of the past. Trapped by worn-out ways of relating to our lives. Basically, trapped in a prison of our own making. Sometimes that prison takes the form of an addiction that drains the life force from us. That prison can consist of drugs or alcohol; it can be an addiction to food, gambling, or sex; it can be some other kind of codependency that is having a damaging effect on our life. Whatever you may be relying on to get through the day, if you're not addressing it head-on, it's taking a toll. To one degree or another, it's negatively impacting the parts of your life that matter most, whether that's your relationships, your work and finances, your health, your romantic life, or your relationship with yourself. Addictions and self-destructive behaviors are obstacles that limit us and keep us from becoming the person we hope to be and living the life we have always wanted to achieve.

Anyone who seeks freedom in one or more of its many different forms is on a recovery journey. The details differ, but we all want freedom from the things that keep us feeling separate — from ourselves and from others. That's the first level of freedom we seek: connection, companionship, and love. Then there's the freedom we seek within our own minds — from patterns of thinking, perceiving, behaving, and interacting that leave us feeling like hamsters on a wheel. Round and round we go, getting nowhere, until we're ready to step off and start the life that is patiently and faithfully waiting for us.

However, once we put negative behaviors aside — whether that's addictive drinking, drug use, eating, sex, or whatever else — we discover that our journey is far from over. In fact, it's only just started. Without addiction, we're left with ourselves. And we may not like what we see. We're left with our own mind, our own thoughts, and often a lot of *questions*.

"How do I make peace with the parts of myself that I
    can't necessarily change?"
"How do I open my eyes — and especially my heart —
    to the parts of myself that are beautiful?"
"How do I consider myself worthy of a bright future
    when I've had such a dark past?"
"How do I even figure out what I want?"
"How do I embrace the totality of who I am? That's just
    a *lot*, isn't it?!"

In other words, a recovery journey is about both what we
stop doing and what we start doing. In order to answer these
difficult questions — about self-acceptance, who we are, and
what we want — we have to develop self-care practices that
allow us to quiet the noise of the world, clear away some of the
internal "clutter," and become present to the life that is being
lived through us. We have to stop hiding and trying to "get it
together" in secret and give ourselves the opportunity to grow
in the sunlight — out in the fresh, open air.

For me, being in recovery from addiction, and cultivating
a self-care practice over time that supports my recovery, has
given me a sense of freedom that I feel every day in my body
and in my mind. Among many other gifts, it has given *me* back
to me. It has been a long yet fruitful process of recovering myself. And that's the kind of freedom that I wish for you.

Inside of addiction, we're under the spell of whatever thing
has a firm grip on us, and we lose ourselves. We have gone
searching outside of ourselves for *something* to make us feel
better — or at least feel okay. Before I picked up my first drink
or drug, I used food to change how I felt. I was not comfortable being Steven. However, outside things only provide

momentary peace from the discomfort we feel from living. And all that outward reaching makes us lose touch with the things that we really need in order to take care of ourselves. That includes how we take care of ourselves physically, how we take care of everyday practical matters, how we take care of our relationships, and how we take care of our own heart and mind. Acts of self-care come in many different forms, but all share a single defining quality: They bring us back to self. They are ways of nourishing the sweetness and light that we are.

From Dancer to Healer

The road back home to ourselves can be a long and winding one, for sure. I share some of those details about myself in the chapters ahead to provide a window into what it can be like and to help show you how I arrived at the place where I am now — teaching movement and meditation practices for care of the self and soul. My recovery journey has been both ordinary and extraordinary, and I'd like to start by sharing how it began.

I was an incredibly shy and sensitive child who grew up in a dysfunctional family that relied upon alcohol, drugs, food, and cigarettes to cope with life. Everyone was severely impacted by trauma, and no one knew how to manage it. My father was a police officer, and my mother was a secretary. My sister and I were and still are very close. I discovered I had a natural talent for dance and theater, and those disciplines saved my life in some ways. By the time I experienced my first drunk at the age of fifteen, I was ready. I needed relief from the realities of my life, which contained a broken home, shame about being gay, and frustrations and confusion about my learning disabilities and my inability to do well in school. I loved the way the cold beers made me feel, but I hated the taste. The buzz from the alcohol made me feel warm, smart, funny, sexy, and energized. My mind was finally able to shut down long enough to give me moments of peace and levity. I chased that feeling over and over for the next fifteen-plus years.

In those years I drank and used drugs to feel better in my own skin and to combat boredom and anxiety. It helped me be social despite my introverted nature. I managed to keep up a daily habit without great consequences until I was twenty-nine years old. By that time, I was unhappy in a relationship that I didn't know how to leave. I also had professional challenges that I felt ill-equipped to handle. Plus, I had familial relationships that created a lot of disharmonies. My answer to just about everything was to check out with substances, suppress my feelings, and avoid reality. By this time, I was lying to my partner, having affairs with coworkers (who were also in relationships), gossiping about others, and spending my money frivolously on anything that would change the way that I felt while sinking into financial debt. I remember in the days leading up to my getting sober, I abruptly paused a singing lesson due to the onset of a cocaine-induced bloody nose. Mortified, I ran into the bathroom, hoping that my instructor didn't notice the fluid running down my face. That's just a glimpse of where my addictions took me.

The day I found sobriety was like any other day and altogether different at the same time. I was hungover as usual, but that day I was broken just enough to be willing to try something new. I was at a turning point. I couldn't imagine my life without drugs and alcohol, but I couldn't envision living one more day with them. I was finally done. I could feel it with every ounce of my being. Even with that certainty, I knew I needed help. I made a fateful call to a sober friend who took me to my first recovery meeting. That was remarkable, and I share more stories from this part of my journey later on. However, as I became alcohol-, drug-, and tobacco-free, I had to figure out who I really was and what I really wanted.

Recovery through Movement

I was a professional dancer for many years in New York. I danced with several small dance companies, which led to jobs at the New York City Opera and the Metropolitan Opera. Eventually I auditioned for musicals and landed a job with Disney's *The Lion King*.

After getting sober, I began to look ahead. I knew that being a professional dancer wouldn't last forever. What else could I do? I enjoyed Pilates and followed an inner prompting to become a Pilates instructor. As I taught at studios around the city, I became even more curious about what else I could learn to help others. This led me to traditional Chinese medicine (TCM), and I decided to become an acupuncturist and doctor of Chinese medicine. Starting graduate school for this course of study was a major demarcation point, as I moved from New York to California and started a whole new life.

Ultimately, I discovered that Chinese medicine wasn't the right path for me, and I dropped out of that program. This was far from an easy decision, and this became a painful and tumultuous time. I still faced many unhealed wounds from my past, and yet dropping out also gave me an important gift: the opportunity to know myself in a profoundly deep way. One thing I realized was that I loved qigong (pronounced: *chi-gung*), which is one of the main branches of TCM. Qigong is a system of movement and breathing exercises — a kind of moving meditation that supports the health of body, mind, and spirit. I somehow knew that qigong was a healing method that would help me greatly in my own recovery and be a technique I could share with others. I had never consciously done energy work before, and it helped me understand the immense power that we all hold within ourselves for healing on every level: physical, emotional, mental, and spiritual.

When I was in active addiction, the only way I knew how to manage or calibrate my energy was to either numb myself if I was feeling too much or go in the opposite direction if I wanted to feel more — adding a little something to take me to that next level. Alcohol, drugs, and cigarettes were my solutions to every problem. That was my energy work back then. Looking back now, I realize that dancing was also a form of energy work for me, even if I didn't understand it that way at the time. It is quite striking how my dancing infused joy, confidence, and peace into my life, akin to a spiritual practice, but the toxicity and darkness of my addictions undermined that magic. No matter how often and how passionately I danced, my inner demons drained me of vital energy until I found sobriety. Then, I began learning how to manage my energy through movement, breath, meditation, and — as I was about to discover — therapeutic touch.

Once I left the Chinese medicine program, I literally went down the hall of that same building and enrolled in a massage program. I found many parallels between traditional Chinese medicine, qigong, and massage, which is yet another form of energy healing. Giving and receiving massages daily was a soothing balm for my body and soul. I also discovered that not only could I help people by laying hands on them, but I could teach others how to help themselves through the simple art of self-massage.

Then my life took a wholly unexpected and happy turn. After several years practicing and instructing others in these healing modalities, I met my husband, Lee Harris, who is a gifted intuitive, motivational speaker, author, and musician. In 2016, Lee gave me the opportunity to travel with him on a teaching tour to Australia, Europe, Canada, and the United States. He was leading one- and two-day workshops and asked me to teach the physical aspects of working with energy using qigong, which was a natural fit. I was incredibly excited to bring my love of qigong to people around the world, and that global tour was the start of a new facet of my career. I began creating wellness content to help people to help themselves, which included creating movement- and meditation-based online courses and videos. One of those online courses was destined to become the book you're now holding in your hands.

As I was creating the curriculum for that course and writing this book, I often wondered if my journey to sobriety and recovery would have even been possible without the tools of qigong, self-massage, and meditation, and how it might have differed if I had found them sooner. I'll never know, but I do know I discovered them when I was ready for them, and they supported me exactly where I was. Wherever you are in your journey, I hope you experience the same thing.

The Gift of Recovery

My life in recovery has been perfectly imperfect. I need to be diligent about my self-care as much now as I did when I first put down drugs and alcohol. For me, the 12 steps of recovery are at the center of my self-care. I recently started doing the steps again with a sponsor I met when I first moved to Southern California. Back then, he clearly had something that I wanted — a quiet strength and sensitivity to life that called to me. Today, he also provides something else I need: the know-how to live in recovery in relationship. He's been married a long time, and I am newly married, and this has presented new challenges. "Life is in session" is one way I like to describe the experience when life humbles me. The schoolroom of life offers an intense curriculum. In working the steps again, I'm taking inventory, putting myself in an intentional place of discovery, and asking myself fundamental questions:

Is this thought, behavior, or choice helping me or harming me?
Is it enhancing or diminishing my sobriety?
Is it moving me closer to a drink, or is it moving me further away from a drink?

As you read this book, reflect on your life and challenges and ask yourself similar questions as you decide what to do. The discussions and practices within these pages provide valuable information, insights, connections, and effective methods to help anyone in recovery, but you have to evaluate what is true and best for you. This book cannot and will not be everything to everyone. I intend it to function as only a small piece of anyone's larger journey of recovery.

In essence, in doing this work for myself, I've found two abiding truisms. One is that recovery is a continual, ongoing process. I know that I can't live my life on yesterday's sobriety. Life doesn't stand still, and I must be awake to whatever is happening today. I need to be as emotionally aware and present in each moment as I can be. This is why I gravitate toward these practices, since they help me focus on right now.

The other is that I *need* structure and community. I need a container for my recovery journey along with the camaraderie and guidance of other people as they, like me, try to live life on life's terms. I need others who can help me answer any questions, doubts, or fears I have about where I am in my journey right now. Those people are like wayshowers — people who embody what we hope to achieve — who help light the path for me.

My hope is that this book will be a wayshower of sorts for you — casting a warm and clarifying light on what you most need for the care of your body and soul at this time in your life. Even though the 12 steps have provided this for me, I have not written this to be a 12-step book. In order to benefit from these practices, you don't need any experience with the 12 steps or its many fellowships — such as Alcoholics Anonymous, Narcotics Anonymous, Overeaters Anonymous, Debtors Anonymous, Co-Dependents Anonymous, and so on. That said, the positive impact and influence of the 12 steps in my life are woven into the DNA of what and how I teach, and these practices support them. Further, throughout this book, I have tried to re-create the sense of community that the 12 steps provide. Several of my recovery friends have graciously agreed to share their experiences, perspectives, strengths, and hopes, and these interviews are threads embedded in the tapestry of this material.

In my experience, the recovery of others often supports our own recovery, even when individual journeys are very different. May you find a similarly open and supportive community within the pages of this book.

How to Use This Book

When I first created the online course that became this book, I vividly remember the *fire* that was ignited in me to share with people all the tools that I had gathered in my years of being sober — along with stories that would be sources of comfort and inspiration. I've discovered that it takes many different elements — resources, a blueprint, and a real sense of community — to take care of oneself and to build a rich life, whether you're in recovery or out of recovery.

In preparation for this journey, I would like to offer a few suggestions. First, and most importantly, put aside the common desire — which tends to arise whenever we embark on something new, especially involving our well-being and happiness — to "do it right." Doing it right could look like pushing yourself to start and finish reading the book in seven days. It could look like pushing yourself to create a daily qigong and meditation practice right away, rather than easing into a rhythm that suits your schedule. In this sense, "doing it right" carries an energy of burden and heavy expectations that can drain the joy out of a new experience. Instead, I encourage you to adopt the 12-step philosophy of "easy does it but do it." Read at a pace that's comfortable. Use the self-massage practices that you find the most helpful or pleasurable. Know that if your day takes an unexpected turn and the time you put in your calendar to meditate or practice qigong needs to be changed, it's okay. Allow yourself to find your own groove with your self-renewal practices.

If you encounter a suggestion, story, or perspective that brings up resistance, see if you can be curious about it rather than quickly rejecting it. In 12-step recovery, coming to a conclusion before you have all the facts — or before you've identified the emotional impact of an experience, event, and so on — is referred to as "contempt prior to investigation." Instead, look at resistance as a signal or messenger, and see if it's offering a meaningful discovery about yourself. For example, if a little resistance bubbles up as you read someone's story, rather than focus on the specific details of the story, see if you can identify the feelings arising in you. You may find that this feeling represents a part of you that simply wants to be acknowledged. The source of resistance may be as simple as that.

That said, with everything I offer here, I invite you to take what you need and leave the rest. At the end of the day, you get to choose which practices, tools, and ideas you accept or reject. But before making any decisions, give yourself a moment to pause, a moment to breathe, and just see what's there. Dipping below the level of thought, what do you find? What feeling, sensation, or need do you make contact with? This kind of intimate self-inquiry is at the heart of the *Recovering You* process.

Tending to the Garden of Your Well-Being: The Practices

One of the promises of recovery, especially 12-step recovery, is that we will get to a point where we experience a genuine sense of happiness, joy, and freedom. But once we achieve that, once we're seated in that place of fulfillment, there is still more to be done. Our highest well-being is like a garden that needs ongoing attention. We have to keep coming back to water, fertilize, prune, and pick the fruits of our labor. Tending to the sacred ground of our own body, mind, and spirit is what self-care is all about.

In this book, I guide you through methods that I know can have a profound impact. I've experienced this in my life and witnessed it in others. The key, however, is incorporating them over time into an ongoing, regular routine. Here are the core elements of *Recovering You*.

Everyday Self-Care

Chapter 1, "Practicing Self-Care during Recovery," describes what a healthy self-care routine looks like and how to build a lasting practice in your own way, at your own pace. Keep this advice in mind as you read the rest of the book, explore the concepts and techniques, and decide what to incorporate on a regular basis, but without trying to do too much and becoming overwhelmed.

This chapter also introduces three important practices that, to me, are essential for daily wellness: deep breathing, self-massage, and meditation. These highly effective techniques don't require any formal training. Not only are they easy to learn and do, they provide an opportunity in almost any moment to be kind and gentle with yourself, which is at the heart of self-care practice.

As I say, when our addictions express themselves, we lose

track of ourselves for a time. Yet what I've discovered over years of practice is that deep breathing, self-massage, and meditation provide opportunities to get back to ourselves — to relieve stress, tension, and pain and remember at the most visceral level who we are and what we need. We don't need to go outside of ourselves to find ourselves. That never works.

Recovery Toolbox

In the rest of the book, each chapter explores a topic that is essential to address for those of us in recovery. These are emotional experiences and states of being — such as fear, shame, isolation, faith, and gratitude. Each chapter also includes a series of sections that help you explore, examine, and work with that issue in your own life. In the "Recovery Toolbox," I provide a range of short exercises that are designed to be quick and easy. Some provide somatic experiences to gain insights through the physical body. Others invite reflection, and others describe specific actions you can take to encourage transformation, alignment, and well-being. All are opportunities to assess where you stand with the concepts each chapter raises while providing concrete steps for moving forward in your recovery journey.

Deep-Diving Discovery Questions

In order to support and deepen your own insights, understanding, and wisdom, each chapter includes a list of reflective questions for you to consider. As you contemplate and respond to these questions, I recommend writing in a journal or notebook.

Writing by hand helps to slow down brain waves, induce calm and presence, and deepen our thinking. That said, if you prefer writing on a computer, that is also fine.

Mindful Movement Moments

Each chapter ends with a short, qigong-based mindful movement. When you finish a chapter, I recommend taking a break from reading and doing this movement before continuing. This will help you feel and acknowledge whatever has arisen while reading. This is especially helpful if difficult or uncomfortable emotions have surfaced, since the movement provides an opportunity to process whatever has come up. Of course, these movements can be done at any time, and if you wish, you can combine some or all into longer routines. I provide further advice on this later in the book.

Each movement is also accompanied by illustrations showing how to do it, and videos can also be found on my website (www.stevenwashingtonexperience.com). If possible, I recommend wearing comfortable, loose-fitting clothing and choosing a place that is relatively free of noise and potential interruption.

Qigong is a brilliant system of movement and breathing exercises that is a revered part of traditional Chinese medicine. The word *qigong* combines the Chinese words for energy ("qi") and work or skill ("gong"). So, the practice of qigong is simply about becoming skillful at managing our own energy, and there are thousands of styles, each as unique as the people who created them.

Since stress and addiction deplete our energy, qigong movements hold a tremendous amount of power to help cultivate and move energy within the body. When done often, they can help increase strength and flexibility as well as calmness of mind. They also free emotional blocks that form because of stress. There are many tools offered in this book, but movement is the pillar of this work. Use the movements to facilitate growth and healing. Some people believe it is necessary to have a vast knowledge of this modality to reap the rewards of it. That is not true. Qigong is medicine for body, mind, and spirit that is available to everyone. Practice the movements and allow the process to unfold wherever you are in your journey.

The Alchemy of Self-Care and Community

Teaching and guiding people through these recovery practices is one of the most incredible journeys of my life. All combined, these methods are a kind of medicine for the soul. There are so many lessons that recovery has taught me about how to enhance our lives, tend to our gardens, and live the best life that we can. And I'm always in search of more tools because life changes all the time. Sometimes what worked yesterday doesn't work today, and that awareness keeps me open to possibilities: *What else can I gather? What else can I discover to help me where I am right now? What else can I learn that will allow me to be a more effective teacher?*

That last question is especially poignant. It reminds me that, as the saying goes, "it takes a village to raise a child." It also takes a village to turn a drunk and an addict around. It takes a village to help an adult live a better life. Self-care and community go hand in hand. They support and foster each other. No one can do life alone, and that's one of the interesting things about addiction. Addiction breeds isolation, placing us on an island all on our own, and recovery is the opposite. In recovery, we get off that island, that place we were shipwrecked, and make our way back to community, to belonging.

For me, one of the greatest gifts of being in recovery is community. I accept all the help that I can get. With that in mind, I've included a Resources section that provides information on various communities and resources you might explore.

Finally, before turning to chapter 1, pause and consider: Where are you today? What's happening around you? What are your plans and priorities? And most importantly, what's happening *inside* of you? How are you feeling? When you ask these questions, what's the first thing that comes to mind? Just acknowledge those answers, which are the essence of your truth in this moment. If you find it hard to get through the day without drinking or drugging or engaging in some other destructive behavior, let this book be a companion to help you to approach life one day at a time. Try as we may, none of us can live more than one day at a time, and we can't do sobriety more than one day at a time either. But if we can string days together into months, and months into years, this one-day-at-a-time approach is how we can build a new, better life.

This book is just one step in your recovery journey. There have been many steps before it, and there will be many after it. Thank you for arriving here with me, inside the sacred container of *Recovering You*. I hope this book inspires you to take good care of yourself and to honor the divine being that you are.

CHAPTER 1

· · · · · · · · · · ·

PRACTICING SELF-CARE
DURING RECOVERY

Self-care is a practice of taking an active role in protecting one's
own well-being and happiness, during periods of stress.

— OXFORD DICTIONARY

In active addiction, the body often takes a backseat to our primal need to satisfy our addiction. I can't tell you how often I've heard recovering alcoholics and addicts say that they neglected the needs of their body while active. Ignoring hunger pains and choosing to drink or drug instead. Disregarding signals from the body that it is full and continuing to eat to satisfy an insatiable emotional hunger. Developing poor hygiene habits because the addiction has taken over. Letting go of physical fitness, or conversely, overexercising to achieve an impossible goal. And lastly, ignoring signs of disease that the body delivers to alert us of health problems. We can lose our way around self-care in active addiction and beyond. After an extended period of neglect, it can be quite daunting to develop good habits around health and well-being.

The process of self-care is a lifelong endeavor, and our commitment to it ebbs and flows. This chapter provides advice for developing and maintaining healthy self-care habits, ones that can be used to incorporate all this book's exercises and practices into your daily routine. It also includes three calming, centering practices — deep breathing, self-massage, and meditation — that are helpful at any time. Doing these on a regular basis can have a profound effect on your recovery and your life, and they can help you integrate the concepts in this book.

There are always periods in our lives when self-care isn't a priority, but today is a new day. Now is the time to take good care of yourself. You are worth it.

Developing Practical, Flexible Self-Care Habits

All the practices in this book are designed to bring balance and harmony to your life, but they only work if you use them regularly, as part of your everyday life. Whatever your goals and past experiences, use these practices as an opportunity to reinvest in your well-being and to slow down and listen to your inner wisdom.

Here are some things to consider when adopting a new self-care regime. First, choose activities that you enjoy, since we have a hard time committing to activities we don't enjoy. I encourage you to try all the ideas in this book at least once, particularly those you've never done before, but if you have other activities that enhance your well-being, do those as well or instead. Listen to your heart.

Next, consider how you will incorporate new practices into your life. For instance, if you like self-massage, think about when you can work it into your day. When would it be easiest or most beneficial to do: in the morning, afternoon, or evening? Plan ahead for when you will do activities, and adjust your current routine to accommodate them. This chapter's self-massage practices are simple and can be done anytime and anywhere. They are most potent when we feel stressed, tense, tired, or uneasy. I also provide multiple techniques for different parts of the body. So, you might find you prefer doing all the techniques at once at a certain time every day, but that isn't necessary. Maybe only one body part feels like it needs regular attention. Or simply let inspiration and intuition be your guide, and do self-massage whenever it feels like it would give you the most benefit in the moment. For instance, I massage my feet most nights before I go to bed. This routine works for me because it allows me to sleep better by relaxing my body and shedding anxiety. Give yourself permission to explore what is best for you.

Deep breathing is another practice that is available anytime, literally twenty-four hours a day, seven days a week. This physiological activity helps build awareness. By paying close attention to how we feel emotionally, we can become conscious of how emotions change our normal breathing, and then how deep breathing can calm and change our emotions. For example, when I was in early recovery, my therapist encouraged me to pay attention to my emotions. When strong ones would pop up, he advised me to pause, place one hand on my heart, and take a few deep breaths. This calmed me and provided some clarity about why I felt whatever I was feeling. Very useful in life and in recovery. Nineteen years later, I still do some version of this. Thus, deep breathing is another short, simple practice that can be done as part of a regular routine, such as first thing in the morning, and also in any moment throughout the day.

At the conclusion of this chapter, I discuss meditation and provide a specific practice. Truthfully, I found that it took a lot of patience and diligence to incorporate meditation into my regular self-care. You may also find that some activities require more work or commitment. That's okay. The benefits are often worth the effort, but we have to build up to them. Know that your self-care practices will grow and change as you become more skilled and comfortable. My meditation practice today doesn't resemble what it looked like in my early years. In the beginning, I meditated only very sporadically. I didn't have much patience for it, and it was important that I allowed it to be that way. What helped me most, though, was that I never completely gave up on trying to do it. Eventually I found a willingness and an approach that worked for me, and this has allowed me to be consistent with it.

Another thing to consider as you construct a new self-care routine is to start small and keep things simple, particularly at first. See if you can do self-massage or deep breathing for only two or three minutes a day, and as you become comfortable with them, increase the time or frequency. The guided meditation at the end of this chapter is meant to take about twenty minutes. If that feels daunting, start by meditating for only five minutes. In addition, for activities that take longer, do them less often. For longer meditations, I recommend choosing one day (or maybe two) per week to be your meditation day. Then schedule half an hour and choose a quiet, comfortable space where you won't be disturbed.

Another activity that can take longer is journaling. Reflective writing takes focused attention, and depending on how involved you get, writing may take anywhere from fifteen minutes to an hour. This requires a bit of planning to make sure that you have quiet, uninterrupted time that doesn't need to be cut short. As you progress through the book, I recommend anticipating the need to set time aside to write about each chapter's topic.

Then, chapters 2 to 9 end with a brief qigong exercise. These should take only five or ten minutes, and I recommend doing them after you read each chapter in order to help integrate the teachings into your body. Of course, I also encourage you to do these movements daily or even several times per day as part of an ongoing self-care routine. Like deep breathing, these movements are especially helpful when strong emotions surface.

Finally, set realistic goals for yourself, and be self-aware of your own reactions as you engage with these practices. If you feel rushed, resistant, or burdened by something, then pull back without completely abandoning the activity. Change the duration and frequency of your practice. Give yourself permission to judge and adjust where you need to.

Typically, it's a good idea to try a new self-care activity or routine for at least seven days, and then reflect on how it makes you feel. If you feel better for having done the practice, you now have firsthand evidence that it works for you, and this can provide the incentive to keep going.

By being gradual, flexible, realistic, and aware, you set yourself up for success.

The Benefits of Breathing

The rest of this chapter presents three practices that are particularly useful whenever you feel upset or overwhelmed. Let's begin with breathing. On average, a person with a healthy respiratory system takes about 12 to 16 breaths per minute, 960 breaths per hour, and 23,040 breaths per day. Thank goodness that the body breathes for us. We don't have to think about breathing because our brains control the act of respiration.

We can learn a lot, however, by paying attention to our breath and tapping into its healing power. By noticing how we're breathing, we can identify how we feel, and by consciously adjusting our breath, we can enhance our overall well-being. When we are at ease, the breath tends to be deeper and slower. When we are stressed and anxious, the breath is often short, sharp, and choppy. Deep breathing exercises an important muscle in the body, the diaphragm. The diaphragm is a dome-shaped muscle in the chest cavity right below the lungs. When we inhale, the diaphragm draws downward, creates a vacuum for the lungs, and draws air into the body. At the exact same time, the intercostal muscles, which are between the ribs, expand to give the lungs space to expand, and the chest muscles and small neck muscles lift the rib cage. Once the lungs are full of air, the diaphragm relaxes and floats upward to push air out of the lungs. And so the dance of breathing continues, again and again and again.

Here are just a few of the benefits that slow, deep breathing provides:

- It activates the parasympathetic nervous system, which stops releasing cortisol, the stress hormone, and starts releasing endorphins, the feel-good hormones.

- It stimulates the lymphatic system and detoxifies the body.
- It increases energy in the body. More oxygen in the blood improves bodily functions.
- It improves digestion as the full movement of the diaphragm muscle massages internal organs.

Breathing with awareness also allows us to be present for the moment we are living in. So often we are living either in the past or in the future. Also, the brain is hardwired to focus on the negative. This defense mechanism is designed to keep us safe from harm, but it can be counterproductive and self-destructive in everyday life. This mechanism can lead us to focus on the past with regret, so we spend our time and energy wishing that we could have said or done something differently or that we could have avoided parts of yesterday. And it can cause us to anticipate the future with fear, rather than hope or excitement — fear that we won't get what we want or that we'll lose what we have or that whatever we're hiding will be found out. We are powerless in the past and the future, but we are powerful in the present. The here and now holds great potential, and deep breathing is the doorway to this potential.

Deep Belly Breathing

Deep belly breathing might be the simplest and most powerful exercise in this book. Either sit, stand, or lie down on your back. Choose the position that is most comfortable for you.

Place the palm of your hand on your abdomen. Take a deep, slow breath in through your nose and allow your abdomen to expand like a balloon. Exhale the breath out through your mouth and allow your abdomen to soften. Be sure to release all the air out before taking your next inhale. On your inhalation, envision drawing pure energy and potential into your body. On your exhalation, imagine releasing tension and worry out of your body and mind. Try to relax the body as much as possible while you breathe. If possible, stretch your inhalation for up to five counts and elongate your exhalation for five counts or more. If that timing doesn't feel right for you, try using four counts for each part of the breath. Do this for up to ten breaths, and when finished, just return to a normal breathing pattern. Notice how you feel.

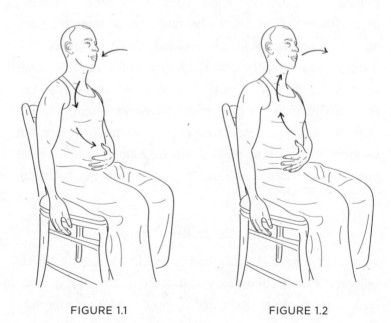

FIGURE 1.1   FIGURE 1.2

The Kindest Gift: Self-Massage

The act of massaging your own body is one of the kindest and most nurturing gifts that you can give yourself. In our active addictions, being kind to the body is not always at the top of our to-do list. So once we are in recovery, it's a good idea to give ourselves the care that we may have deprived ourselves of previously.

One of the best experiences of my life was being a student in massage school. Before that, I had always enjoyed massage and knew the power that it held, but while in school, I learned why it felt so good and what it was doing for me physiologically. Using our hands to press and rub our skin and underlying muscles can relieve tension and pain in the body, which is often a byproduct of stress. We all experience stress, and some amount is healthy. However, too much stress is problematic. Life in early recovery and beyond can be overwhelming and disorienting. Taking a few minutes each day to tend to key parts of the body can be impactful.

In this practice, I focus on the hands, feet, and ears. Traditional Chinese medicine proposes that the vastness and wonder of nature and the universe are mirrored in the human body. The microcosm reflects the macrocosm. The same is believed true for the human body, in which the whole is mirrored in the hands, feet, and ears. In this ancient medical tradition, massaging or inserting acupuncture needles in specific body parts can affect the entire body. By massaging our feet, we can relieve pain and tension not only in the feet but in other parts of the body. By massaging our hands, we can help reduce stress. By massaging our ears, we can relax the entire body and self-regulate. After all, when we are acting out addictively, somewhere in our motivation is the desire or goal to change how we feel. We want to alter our physical and emotional state and ultimately regulate our emotions. Through the self-care practice of self-massage, we can naturally alter our physical and mental state. We can unlock the healing power within by turning off our body's stress response and activating the part of our nervous system that naturally releases the feel-good hormones that make us feel calm, relaxed, and energized.

In the illustrations that follow, I map each body part to show how massage can affect the entire body. I offer this as a general guide, but it's not necessary to adhere to these in a strict manner. By intuitively massaging and listening to your body and what it desires, you will navigate the magnificent parts of yourself with ease. Think of the maps as trail guides, and use them as much or as little as you'd like on your somatic adventure.

Foot, Hand, and Ear Massage

Let's begin with the feet. Each foot has up to twenty-six bones, thirty joints, and more than a hundred muscles, tendons, and ligaments that work together to provide support, balance, and mobility. Our feet are the most used and abused parts of the body. They carry us around from place to place and sometimes in ill-fitting shoes. They deserve our attention and care. In the foot reflexology graphics on pages 31 and 32, notice how every part of the body is represented on the soles of the feet. From the heels all the way up to the toes are sections that correspond with the pelvis, nerves, organs, spine, sinuses, and brain. The microcosm mirrors the macrocosm.

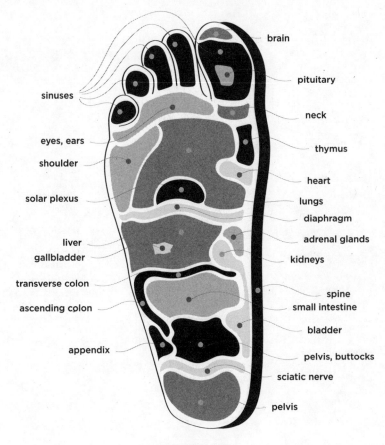

FIGURE 1.3A

There are several ways to approach foot massage. One simple technique is using a small ball to massage the foot. From a seated or standing position, place on the floor a tennis ball (or any other ball that's comparable in size). Place your foot over the ball, starting anywhere you would like. Apply a comfortable pressure and gently roll the ball forward and back along the entire length of your foot. Pay attention to any tender spots. If you happen to find one, pause and allow the ball to add static pressure to that spot. Breathe deeply, notice the sensations, and

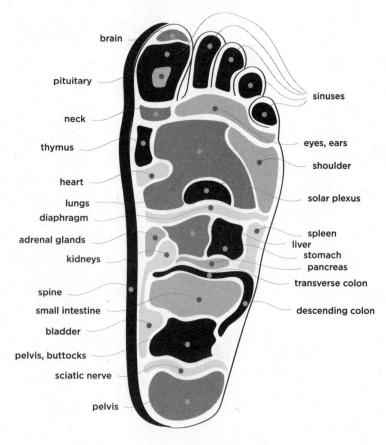

FIGURE 1.3B

keep doing this for at least thirty seconds or up to one or two minutes. Observe if the sensations change. You may notice that the tenderness dissolves, or you may become aware of something else. From there, move to another tender spot and repeat the process.

Another foot massage technique is done with the hands. From a seated position, cross one ankle over one knee and hold your foot in both hands. With your thumb pads, incrementally rub up and down the length of your foot. Again, search for a tender or tense spot. If you find one, pause and apply static pressure with the tips of your thumbs. Breathe deeply throughout and notice what you feel. Observe the sensations in your foot and notice if any changes take place. Remember to use a pressure that is comfortable for you. It is also effective to hold the top of the foot with one hand and use the knuckles of the other hand to massage the sole of the foot. Pulling the toes and pinching them are great as well.

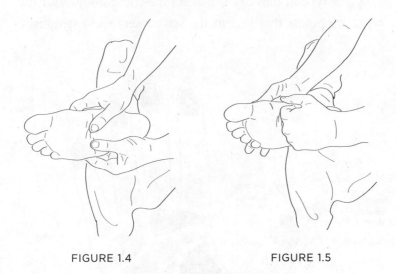

FIGURE 1.4   FIGURE 1.5

When you finish massaging one foot, do the other. One way to make the experience extra special is to use your favorite lotion or scented massage oil. This will give your strokes a lovely and easy glide; it isn't necessary to use a great deal of it. A little goes a long way. Once you've completely massaged both feet, close your eyes and rest for a moment. Notice how your feet and entire body feel after this brief self-care practice. Take a few deep breaths and witness the sensations, as well as your mental and emotional state.

Next let's work on the hands. The human hand is made up of the wrist, palm, and fingers and consists of twenty-seven bones, twenty-seven joints, thirty-four muscles, over a hundred ligaments and tendons, and many blood vessels and nerves. The hands do a great deal for us, and it is important to take care of them. As we age, we tend to lose strength and flexibility in the hands. Regular hand massages are a great practice to adopt.

Like the foot reflexology chart, the hand chart below shows how this type of massage can affect the entire body. Near the wrist are points that benefit the sciatic nerve and lymphatic

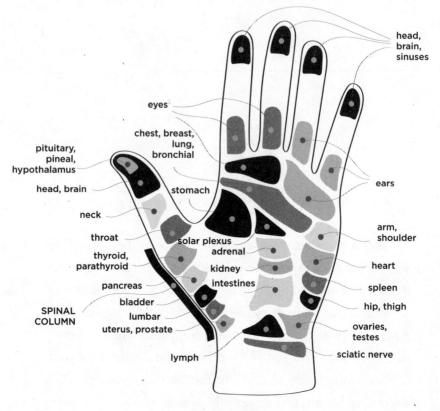

FIGURE 1.6A

system. Organ systems can be accessed through the palm of the hand. The spinal column can be affected by massaging the thumb. Lastly, the head, brain, and sinuses are treated by working on the fingertips. The macrocosm in the microcosm.

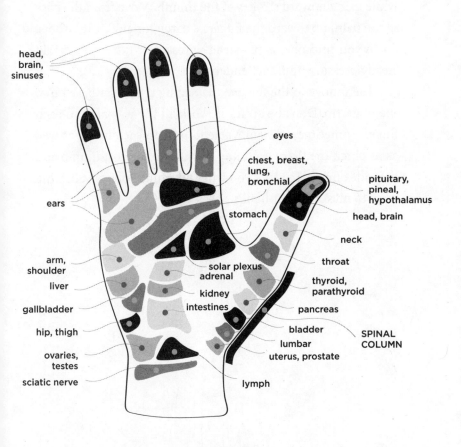

FIGURE 1.6B

As with the feet, you don't have to follow the illustration when massaging your hands. I encourage you to use your intuition during this self-care practice, but here are a couple of techniques to explore. The first method is to hold one hand in the palm of the other hand while the palms face upward. Use the support hand as your tool. Four fingers of the support hand hold the other hand in place while you massage the palm with your thumb. Again, use a pressure that is comfortable for you while using upward strokes of the thumb. Move from the base of the palm up toward the fingers. Search for any tender spots. Once you find one, apply steady pressure to that spot. Hold steady pressure until the tenderness subsides.

Then move to the fingers, massaging the finger base up to the fingertip. Don't be afraid to work all the way around each finger. Sometimes it is enjoyable to pull on each finger as well as to pinch the tip of each finger with the support thumb and the index finger. I'm sure you will find a multitude of satisfying ways to massage your hands.

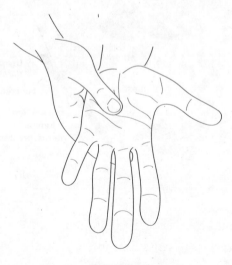

FIGURE 1.7

Another technique that I recommend is to sit in a chair and rest the back of one hand on the top of one thigh. Allow the hand to relax on the thigh. Make a soft fist with the other hand, and applying a comfortable pressure, rub your knuckles along the resting palm on your thigh. Begin near the wrist and rub the knuckles upward toward the base of your fingers. Again, search for any tender spots, and apply steady pressure until the tenderness subsides. You could also switch tools here and use your thumb again to apply steady, deep, focused pressure on your target location. This could all be done with dry hands, but applying some sort of cream or oil improves the glide of your strokes and gently moisturizes your hardworking hands.

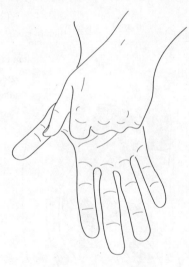

FIGURE 1.8

Once you have massaged both hands, take a moment to rest and observe the sensations in your hands. Observe what you feel in your entire body. Notice your breathing. Are you able to breathe deeply after this self-care practice? I certainly hope so.

Finally, let's explore the ears. The outer ear is called the auricle. It is essentially made of cartilage, skin, and over five hundred nerve endings. Ear massage or reflexology is an effective form of self-care for the entire body and for the emotions. This is helpful for anyone managing depression, sadness, worry, anxiety, or anger. These are all emotions that everyone faces in everyday life, but they arise especially for those of us recovering from any form of addiction or trauma.

In the graphic below, notice that every part of the body is represented in the ear. Points at the base of the ear correspond with the head, and points at the top of the ear relate to the feet and fingers.

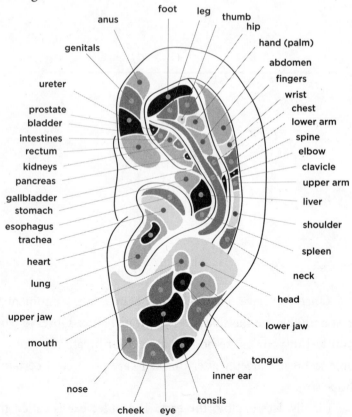

FIGURE 1.9

To begin, I recommend briskly rubbing your hands together to create heat. Fifteen to thirty seconds should be enough to energize your hands before you touch your ears. Make sure that you are comfortable, whether standing, sitting, or lying down. Cup your hands and gently place them over your ears. Allow your ears to absorb the warmth of your hands for a moment or two. Take a few deep breaths. With your fingertips, begin to gently squeeze the tops of your ears. While you squeeze, softly pull up and out, forward and back. From there, squeeze specific points between the thumbs and index fingers, working your way from the outer edges of the ears toward the ear canal. Eventually, work your way down to the lobes of the ears. It is a delicious feeling to pull the lobes down and out.

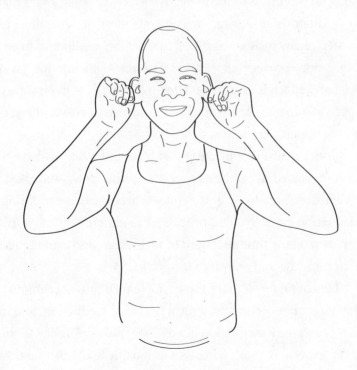

FIGURE 1.10

Once you've completed your ear massage, allow the hands to rest on your lap or by your sides. Observe what you feel. Notice the sensations in your ears. You may feel heat, warmth, tingling, or perhaps something else. Just be a witness. Also notice your emotional state. Perhaps you are calmer now than before, or perhaps that tiny worry that had your attention earlier in the day has faded away. Perhaps your thoughts are less frenetic. You have cultivated a moment of peace. Enjoy it and know that you can always return to moments like this whenever you need to.

Meditation: Space to Reflect

What does it mean to meditate? Webster's dictionary says that to meditate is to engage in contemplation or reflection. In 12-step recovery, it is suggested that we use meditation to enhance our recovery experience. The act of meditating gives time and space to our lives. Time to reflect in a neutral way. Space to allow inner wisdom and guidance to rise to the surface of our consciousness.

I once heard in a meeting that meditation doesn't have to be complicated. It can be as simple as sitting down and taking several deep breaths while the coffee is brewing in the morning. Meditation can also be a process of reading inspiring words and then taking time afterward to sit, breathe, and contemplate their meaning and relevance to your life.

I encourage you to try these simple meditative techniques. But another, more-involved form is guided meditation, and in 2018, I created a meditation titled "Sober Soldier." Today, I look at my experience with addiction as a battle and a blessing. At times, I felt like I was in a war between my lower and higher selves, but it has all been a blessing because I've learned so much about myself and the world, and it has given me the opportunity to build a rich spiritual life.

To do this meditation, first find a quiet place where you can be alone and take an inward journey. Then, you can either read the meditation to yourself from the book, or access a free recorded version of the meditation on my website (www.stevenwashingtonexperience.com). Either way, let the words wash over you, and once the meditation is over, be still. Take a few deep breaths and reflect. Trust the insights or peace you encounter during this time. It is all here to serve you.

• Sober Soldier Meditation •

Welcome to your meditation. I invite you to sit or lay in a comfortable position. Allow your feet to be firmly planted on the floor and your hands to rest on your lap or at your sides. I invite you to close your eyes and relax into this position and allow your chair, cushion, mat, or bed to support you.

Take a deep breath into your body. And exhale the air out of your body. Witness the cycles of your breath. Take a moment to watch your breath without judgment. Notice the release throughout your body as you breathe in and out. Every breath is fortifying your physical and inner life. You are strong, supported, blessed, sober, open, loved, and connected to a Power greater than yourself. A Power that knows and accepts you for who you are. Breathe in the love, acceptance, and grace. I invite you to allow this love, acceptance, and grace to wash over you like water.

Imagine yourself standing in a beautiful grotto beneath a waterfall on a warm summer day. The sun is bright and shines through the trees in dazzling ways. The water is warm and washes over you. The water flows from your head, down your face, and along your neck, and trickles down your arms to your fingertips. Tiny drops of water fall from your fingertips to the water surrounding your legs and feet. Notice the sensation of water streaming down your torso to your legs and into the supportive, cleansing water that surrounds you. You are safe, strong, supported, blessed, sober, open, loved, and connected to a Power that is greater than yourself. Take a deep breath in and out. Notice what may be a deep level of peace, relaxation, confidence, and trust within you that all is well in this moment. You have everything you need right here, right now.

Allow the words of this peaceful prayer to infuse peace and strength into your body, mind, and spirit.

Lord, make me a channel of thy peace.
That where there is hatred, I may bring love.
That where there is wrong, I may bring a spirit of
   forgiveness.
That where there is discord, I may bring harmony.
That where there is error, I may bring truth.
That where there is doubt, I may bring faith.
That where there is despair, I may bring hope.
That where there are shadows, I may bring light.
That where there is sadness, I may bring joy.
Lord, grant that I may seek rather to comfort than to be
   comforted.
To understand than to be understood.

To love than to be loved.
For it is by self-forgetting that one finds.
It is by forgiving that one is forgiven.
It is by dying that one awakens to Eternal Life.

Take a deep breath into your body and then release it.

As we bring this guided meditation to a gentle close, I invite you to wiggle your toes and fingers and stretch your body any way that it intuitively would like to move. Gently open your eyes and take in what you see before you.

I hope that you enjoyed this meditation and that we share another one together very soon. Many blessings.

CHAPTER 2

. . . .

UNDERSTANDING ISOLATION

But there are other words for privacy and independence.
They are isolation and loneliness.

— MEGAN WHALEN TURNER, *THE KING OF ATTOLIA*

It happens gradually. Sometimes imperceptibly. The world gets smaller and smaller as we retreat into the habits, feelings, thoughts, and places that feel "safe" — comfortable in the old-shoe sort of way. Loss, trauma, and pain of all kinds can initiate the gradual separation that erodes the connection between ourselves and others. For those in addiction, the isolation can easily move to extremes. My recovery friend Randee is a married, seventy-five-year-old writer with double-digit sobriety. She is a voice in recovery that I trust, and I asked her what isolation looked and felt like to her in active addiction.

"Well, it looked like a blackout," she said. "It's kind of the ultimate isolation because you don't have to remember what you did. I recall being at an open house for my kids, and I just wanted to go home and drink. I couldn't wait to get out of there. I felt like I wasn't a good enough mom. I kept feeling all these things that were driving me to want to get away from the other parents at the school, who I was imagining as having absolutely no problems."

Untreated alcoholism has the power to distort one's thinking and allow an individual to believe that they're the only person with life problems in a large, crowded room. Everyone has problems, but the person struggling with addiction uses their substance as a "solution" to their troubles.

When I reflect on my own story, I can identify a pattern of isolation that is a distinct part of me, one that began long before I ever picked up a drink, a drug, or a cigarette. When I was between the ages of five and ten, I had a recurring dream of being trapped and alone in a deep, dark well. As I looked up toward the light of the sky, I saw the silhouette of another person. That person was me looking down at myself in the well — completely powerless to change the unfortunate circumstance. As a child, I couldn't understand the symbolism of the dream, but as a recovered alcoholic and addict who has been to hell and back, I now see how the dream foreshadowed future suffering and the opportunity to rise above it.

Randee shared her experience as a child. "I felt very isolated as a kid. I felt like everybody else's family was perfect and mine was weird — because of where I lived at the time, and everything, really. But I think everyone feels that their family is weird."

Much like Randee, I didn't feel as though I had much in common with other children. I couldn't see how they could possibly identify with my world. Our worlds seemed so disparate. I perceived that others had better lives than mine based on what my eyes could see. Comparison is such a precarious thought process. It steals our joy. Most often, comparison leaves us holding the short end of the stick. Randee agreed:

"I guess isolation also is comparing myself to other people and just putting myself down. It's like thinking, *I am not good enough to be here.*"

No matter how the pattern begins, isolation and addiction go hand in hand. The addicted person wants nothing more than to be alone with the thing that they are addicted to, the substance or behavior. It's almost like having an itch that we can't help but scratch. Through the process of isolation, the world of the addicted person becomes smaller and smaller until they are separate and alone in the ways that allow them to continue using. In my days of drinking, I would commiserate with others at bars or parties, but I couldn't wait to get home and drink with impunity. I often hear others describe the same or similar behavior when they are active in their addiction.

Causes of Isolation

Although patterns of isolation are usually multilayered, I've discovered that there are three main reasons why people isolate: to avoid conflict, to hide shame, and to relinquish control. Let's look at each one carefully.

Avoiding Conflict

Someone isolates because they want to avoid conflict. Their friends and family care about them and want them to heal, have a better life, and stop the addictive behavior. The person, however, is caught in a vicious cycle: As they express the addiction and perform the addictive behaviors, they must build walls around them to escape the suggestions and pleas of their family and friends to stop.

I recall a period around 2001 when I was living in Toronto. I had a partner at that time, and we were separated due to our professional commitments. He was traveling with a touring show across the United States, and I had just begun a new job dancing in a Broadway show. I had already crossed that invisible line from using alcohol recreationally to doing so in a very addictive way. I had started using cocaine frequently as well. I remember avoiding phone calls from my partner, and I wouldn't call him as frequently as he wanted. Often, I wouldn't answer the phone when he called because I knew he would be able to tell that something was off. All of this clearly bothered him, and he sensed that I was lying.

Lying is an integral part of isolating behavior. I lied to my partner quite a bit during that time. I lied about my drinking and drug use. I lied about who I was spending time with. And I kept pushing him away to avoid conflict. My addictive behavior became a priority for me. I kept him at bay to avoid difficult conversations, but these were inescapable. You can run, but you can't hide forever.

Hiding Shame

Another reason someone isolates is to hide their shame. While we all feel a certain amount of shame as human beings, for those in active addiction, shame accumulates and becomes toxic. It's often shame that we grew up with and now bear the weight of in adulthood. For adults burdened by soul-breaking shame and without the tools to free themselves from it, shame is crippling. Some disguise the shame that lives beneath their skin, but there comes a point when it inevitably expresses itself through addictive behaviors. Shame begets shame, and a relentless cycle begins. Shame feeds the addictive behavior, and the behavior feeds the shame.

In chapter 4, I explore the topic of shame in more detail and look at ways to move past that emotion.

Relinquishing Control

The third primary reason people isolate is because the addiction is running the show. In 2001, when I was avoiding conflict with my partner, I had lost the choice as to whether I was going to drink. It was beyond my control. I had an itch, and I had to scratch it. Alcohol and drugs made the decisions for me. My compulsion was the director, and I was the actor. It was telling me what to do, when to do it, and how to do it. Intoxicating substances ruled me. That's what happens when addiction sets in. Whatever someone's poison is, whether it's alcohol, drugs, gambling, food, sex, a codependent relationship, or something else, addiction is in full swing when any of those things begin to call the shots.

Isolating ourselves to avoid conflict, to hide shame, or because our power of choice is now in the hands of the craving that's wreaking havoc in our lives is a predictable progression of the addictive process. These behaviors come together to create a dynamic that negatively influences the whole of our lives. The cost is high. The self-confidence, self-esteem, and self-love that get decimated in this process are only part of the terrible price we pay.

But in time, what is lost can be found and rebuilt again. There are ways out of isolation. There are solutions to this problem.

Randee, being wise, shared this advice for anyone who is struggling with isolation:

> There is nothing like prayer. But I would try to be more specific than just "God help me." I would be clear and direct. "God, I know you've put people around me that can help me break out of this. Help me to recognize them." And then I would step back and be very vigilant about who those people may be. You know, we are such pessimists as drunks. Somebody smiles at us, and we go straight to "They are probably smiling at somebody behind me. Or it's probably a scam. They want to draw me in and take my money." We usually don't trust the good things that happen. So, I would add to that prayer what you need for someone to be like to help you break out of isolation. Then look around you. And look through the eyes of optimism about life. Make your prayer a request to help you make your life better.

If you are someone who struggles with the concept of God, a Higher Power, or Universal Energy, I want to emphasize that you don't need to embrace any spiritual concept to do this work. It's okay to be where you are with this subject (I explore this further in chapter 9). However, I encourage you to try prayer anyway, even if you don't believe. As Randee describes, prayer can be a visualization tool that helps us identify and focus on what we need and then look for it. When we are desperate for healing, anything that gets our mind focused on positive solutions can help. I know people whose lives have been saved repeatedly by prayer, even though they aren't religious. They got on their knees anyway and prayed to a God they don't believe in, and this helped them feel more connected and less isolated. Praying is an exercise in going beyond the bounds of belief and stepping into the unknown. In prayer, we have nothing to lose, and only something to gain.

Recovery Toolbox

Here are some recovery tools that can be effective ways to avoid isolation and increase communion with others. Try them and see if they have a positive impact on your life.

Call It Out

Naming what you are feeling is an effective way to reduce and regulate the emotions that arise within. There is power in calling out difficult feelings. Suppressing emotions never provides positive results. The feelings get pushed down temporarily and eventually express themselves in negative and unhelpful ways. Naming your dominant emotions is empowering. It allows you to take more control and ownership over your circumstances and moves you toward actions that can transform how you feel. Take a moment right now to check in with yourself; take inventory of your current emotional state. If you are feeling isolated, lonely, or any other heavy emotion, call it out. Make a regular practice of acknowledging your feelings.

Set an Intention to Connect

An intention guides our actions to achieve a certain outcome. To move away from isolation, set an intention to connect more with other people. That's all. Every morning, without knowing exactly what you will do, set that intention, which has the power to inspire and guide your actions. Perhaps you will make a phone call, attend a support group meeting, arrange a coffee date with a friend or loved one, or send a heartfelt email. The specifics don't really matter. By reinforcing our intention to connect, we help keep ourselves on track to transform our life when we feel nervous, self-conscious, or afraid to move beyond our comfort zone.

If you want to have meaningful exchanges with others, deepen your relationships, and feel more connected to humanity, take a few deep breaths and set that intention now. From there you will naturally find ways to do so over time.

Actively Seek Social Connections

Sometimes, when we feel lonely or isolated, we expect or hope that other people will notice and reach out to us. But it is important to take the initiative and reach out first. Don't wait for someone else to make contact. Be proactive and contact them. Taking action, all by itself, can change how we feel. An old recovery slogan that captures this dynamic is "You can't think your way into right action, but you can act your way into right thinking."

Paradoxically, the friendship, fellowship, and connection that we abandon when isolating is all we need to solve the problem. Each of these can be found and cultivated in various ways. What worked best for me as I was getting sober were recovery meetings. They made it possible for me to interact and connect with people who were on a similar journey. As I listened to their stories, I regained strength and hope and gathered information about what I could do next to further break out of the cycle of isolation that I had lived with for so long.

Randee beautifully described to me what it was like when she first started attending meetings:

> Well, it's funny because I felt like I was in a room where I didn't know the language. I was trying to be hip, slick, and cool in the room. I was trying to say something that would make me stand out as somebody who is worthy of attention and friendship, but I didn't know the language. You know? And that was the thing — when I finally got into the program, I knew the language. I was in a meeting the other day and some person said, "Well, I have four days." I know that language now. I know exactly what that means — four days. Oh my God.

Take a moment now to decide how you will reach out if you are feeling isolated or lonely. Decide if you will search for a recovery meeting, whether in-person or online. Or decide which person you will call or write to. Taking action and making contact will certainly help you, and it may help someone else.

Move Your Body

Feelings of isolation and loneliness are intertwined with overall well-being. When people become entrenched in prolonged cycles of loneliness, they tend to create a very small world for themselves without much physical activity. According to the Mayo Clinic, lack of physical activity can lead to depression and anxiety as well as a host of other health problems. On the other hand, consistent exercise combats all these things. It doesn't just help improve high blood pressure, diabetes, and arthritis — it improves our mood, reduces stress, and minimizes loneliness and depression.

This book is founded on the principle that movement and exercise provide emotional and mental benefits. This is why I encourage you to do the qigong exercises when you reach them at the end of each chapter. These are wonderful opportunities to mindfully move your body. And keep these simple exercises handy whenever feelings of isolation and depression arise. By the end of this book, you will have a complete qigong routine to rely upon for support.

In general, I encourage you to regularly incorporate physical activity of all kinds into your life. Take a moment now to create a list of two or three activities that you enjoy and can envision doing daily or at least several times per week. Then set realistic goals that incorporate more movement in a gradual way. Deciding to go to the gym seven days a week, when you don't go at all now, isn't a good way to start. For instance, after work, simply go for an extended walk to take your mind off your worries and increase the opportunity to have social interactions with other people. Don't underestimate the power of a friendly smile, a wave, or a shared hello with someone in your neighborhood. This alone can momentarily lift you out of loneliness and isolation.

Practice the Power of Touch

Yet another way to break free from isolation is through body-work. As a trained massage therapist, I've witnessed the power of touch and know its ability to dissolve emotional and energetic walls. When living an isolated life, people not only lose emotional contact with others, but they lose the nurturing and caring physical contact others provide. The power of touch can do so much to help us remember that we're not alone. There is tenderness and support available to us right there on a massage table. The self-massage practices in this book are effective for this, too, but I also recommend finding a skilled bodyworker or massage therapist in your local area. Ask your friends and family for referrals, which are often a good and safe place to begin.

• **Deep-Diving Discovery Questions** •

I hope that your heart and mind have been stirred by this conversation on isolation. Now I suggest taking some time to reflect on how this issue relates to your life by journaling your answers to the following questions. Ideally, this guided self-inquiry will increase your awareness of these issues and help foster insights and solutions that provide greater freedom from isolation, as well as from the loneliness, avoidance, shame, and lack of control that often accompany these feelings.

1. How often do you spend time alone?
2. Do you feel lonely during these times, or do you welcome the solitude?
3. When you are alone, what do you do with that time?

4. Is there any part of you that is afraid to interact with people? If so, describe how you might soothe the part of you that is afraid.

5. What could you say to this part of you to make reaching out to others easier?

6. If you lived a less-isolated life, what would that look like to you? Where would you go? What would you do? Who would you spend time with?

7. Name all the things you love about life.

8. How can you engage with those things that you love over the next week?

9. Are you willing to commit to taking action — to put that engagement in motion?

• Mindful Movement Moment: •
Pulling Down the Sky

Before reading further, to integrate the teachings of this chapter into your body, mind, and spirit, take a few moments to do this simple qigong exercise called "Pulling Down the Sky." As you do it, call to mind whatever came up for you as you read this chapter, whether that's related to recovery, isolation, or events in your own life. The purpose of this exercise is to calm the mind, relax the body, and anchor you. As you repeat the exercise, it will draw you back to the present moment — where great potential for growth and peace resides.

Ultimately, I've ordered all eight qigong exercises in this book so that, when done together, they make a short, effective qigong routine, one that might take twenty minutes or so, depending on your pace. The first three exercises (in chapters 2 to 4) can be thought of as preparation for the last five (in chapters 5 to 9), which are known as the Five Element Flow. That said, my hope is that you won't approach these exercises in a rigid way. Each can be done alone, and they can be rearranged in various combinations. Explore these movements in whatever ways work best for you, and reap the benefits of them at any time.

1. Start by standing with your legs about shoulder-width apart.
2. As you ground yourself in this position, envision waves of calm gently washing over you (Fig. 2.1).
3. Soften your knees, lengthen your spine, and lift the crown of your head toward the sky. As you do this, allow your arms to be long and relaxed at the sides of your body.

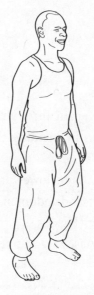

FIGURE 2.1

4. Take a deep inhale through your nose as you lift your arms out to the sides and then up above your head. Gaze upwards as your arms lift (Figs. 2.2, 2.3).

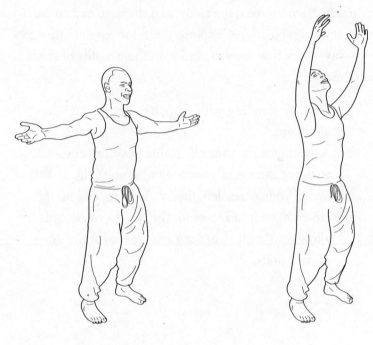

FIGURE 2.2   FIGURE 2.3

5. As you exhale, again through the nose, let your arms float down by bending the elbows outward (Fig. 2.4).
6. Allow your hands to lower and pass in front of your head, heart, and abdomen. Gaze downward as your arms lower (Fig. 2.5).
7. Repeat this exercise at least twelve times.

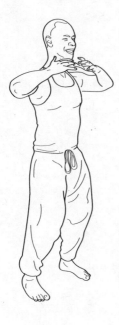 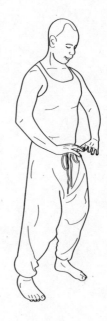

FIGURE 2.4   FIGURE 2.5

• Movement Tips •

- Palms face upward as arms lift.
- Palms face downward as the arms lower.
- Be sure to relax the hands and shoulders through-out.
- Be mindful of releasing excess tension in the shoulders when the arms are above the head.
- Take your time. Coordinate the breath with the movement.
- Listen to your body. Modify when you need to.

CHAPTER 3

. . . .

BEYOND FEAR

Many of our fears are tissue-paper-thin,
and a single courageous step would carry us
clear through them.

— BRENDAN FRANCIS

This chapter explores a part of ourselves that we usually keep well hidden: our fears. Without a doubt, it takes courage to face our fears, to be willing to look beneath the surface and examine what we normally avoid. When we do, we shine a light into the darkness and truly see what's there. Change alone can incite fear. So, to succeed at recovery, and to improve our self-care, we need to examine any resistance or negative responses to recognize and acknowledge the fears beneath them.

My recovery friend Bill and I met in 2017 while at a meeting. Bill is a writer in his early sixties. He has double-digit sobriety and is devoted to helping other people in recovery. I asked him what he thought was the truth about fear.

He said, "It's interesting to look at how we can get caught up in fear, when 90 percent of the time what we worry about never happens."

Fear and addiction go hand in hand. When we feel fear, it's not uncommon for us to have the desire to numb ourselves, to check out or distract from what we are afraid of. Overcoming addiction and having a meaningful life and recovery will always be out of reach unless we find a way to manage our fears when they arise.

Fear is a natural response to any perceived threat. Fear has the potential to keep us safe. It's our instinctive reaction to any potential danger, but it doesn't matter if that danger is real or not. Any threat can cause us to feel fear, and that fear often triggers our "fight, flight, or freeze" response and a sense of panic. Obviously, this affects our ability to make decisions. Fear can interrupt the brain's ability to regulate emotions and read the verbal and nonverbal cues of others or the environment. Fear can lead us to respond to life inappropriately due to our inability to clearly and accurately interpret the information we receive.

Bill shared an early lesson about fear: "Fear can stack up on itself. One on top of the other. My fears led me to develop anxiety, and at the age of twelve I discovered that alcohol would take away the fear and a joint would alleviate my anxiety."

I hope this chapter helps you understand fear and, using the tools provided, learn to navigate this dark territory, manage it better, and move beyond it. Freedom awaits on the other side of fear and worry.

Sharing Fears Helps Eliminate Fear

Sometimes people believe that their fears are unique or that no one else could possibly understand exactly why they are afraid.

Truthfully, we are all afraid of something. It does not matter who we are. No one gets through this life without traversing the complicated road of fear. Everyone has the responsibility of managing their emotions, either with or without prowess. It can be helpful to hear others speak about their fears. Doing so allows us to identify with and acknowledge our shared humanity and struggles. Sharing fears is a window of opportunity that helps us move past our perceptions about someone's inner life just by looking at their external circumstances. We get a chance to see that we are all afraid of the same stuff.

Think about a neighbor or work colleague who seems perfectly put together. They always dress well, stay fit, excel at their job, and have the ideal family. They appear to have it all and wear a smile on their face most of the time. Looks can be deceiving. Unbeknownst to you, they might drink till they're drunk every day without fail. They make excuses to themselves to justify their drinking, but deep down they know there is a problem and they are afraid to stop. They are also afraid to let anyone know, so they project a false image. They want others to think they are perfect out of fear that, if people knew they weren't, they would be rejected.

In this example, several fears are at play. First, there is the fear of not drinking. Many alcoholics and addicts get to a point where they can't imagine continuing along the path of destruction they are on, and yet they can't imagine a life free of what binds them. That was my experience. Second, there is the fear of being seen for who they are. Allowing others to see us in our entirety, flaws and all, is difficult to do. Lastly, there is the fear of being rejected by others. No one wants to be shunned or looked down upon, and we go to all sorts of lengths to avoid it. Hiding addictive or negative behavior is almost always experienced as a necessity for this reason.

These are relatively common fears. I have experienced them and felt them amplified and perpetuated by my addictive behavior, and perhaps you have, too. Here are a few more fears I have navigated in my life:

- Fear of the unknown
- Fear of financial insecurity
- Fear of failure and humiliation
- Fear of success
- Fear of illness and death
- Fear of dying alone
- Fear of abandonment
- Fear of not being loved
- Fear of losing a loved one
- Fear of losing what I have or not getting what I want

I feel certain that all people can find parts of themselves in the list above. And maybe you could add a few more fears to the list as well. Again, I find it comforting and reassuring to know the challenges other people face, particularly those who have intimately experienced the same fears I have. For me, this knowledge creates a sense of community and shared burdens. I feel better about myself and not so alone. Bill discovered this truth for himself: "What I have learned from my fears is that I experience them to develop self-love. I had to break through fears by steadily moving forward, and on the other side was more self-love."

I asked Bill if he had other advice for someone who is overcome by fear and needs help shifting out of that emotion. He said:

Find something in your life that helps you feel grounded, that makes you feel like you are one with the universe, in a way. Whether it is a dog or cat, going into nature, reading a book that makes you feel good, listening to a certain song or meditating to get you to a certain place where you are sitting on a beach, even if you are not on a beach. Those types of things help us realize that the fear is an illusion. I like the saying that fear stands for "false evidence appearing real." Most of our fears are in our heads. Just because I am feeling it doesn't mean it is true. This too shall pass. In my experience, I know that I'm an adult but that doesn't mean I am never afraid. As an adult I need to know that I can take certain actions to feel better and that I innately know this truth.

Recovery Toolbox

Here are some tools that can help you develop a sense of freedom, courage, and more self-love to bolster your recovery. Use them anytime you struggle with fear to help you along your path.

Be Curious: Walk Through Your Fears

A valuable tool I've learned is to be curious about the things that frighten me. I find it is beneficial to "unpack" my fears, one by one, when they arise. In early recovery, when I felt triggered or fearful, I was advised to "play the tape" through to the end. That is, I was encouraged to walk myself through my worst-case scenario and imagine what might happen if my fears became a reality.

Bill expressed a similar sentiment: "I still have a lot of fears today, and at twenty-one years clean and sober, I just learned I have to walk through it. I don't like feeling it, but if I can remember I need to be comfortable being uncomfortable, then when I walk through it, I end up feeling a sense of relief and release."

As an example, I'll unpack one of my fears from my list: my fear of abandonment. This fear has been with me most of my life, and it probably stems from growing up in a broken home. Today, when something triggers that fear — when I become afraid or anxious that someone I care about will leave me — whispers of that old wound surface and inform my reaction. Some small part of me believes I will be alone similar to how I felt abandoned as a child. And hidden within this fear is a deeper fear that, if this person leaves, I will be unable to care for myself and maybe even unable to survive. So what would happen if this person left? As I unpack this worst-case scenario, and I search my life for evidence of my inability to take care of myself, connect with others, and move forward, I can honestly find no evidence of that. The fear is just fear; it's unrealistic, and even a lie. Recognizing this gives me a new perspective and changes my relationship to whatever I was afraid of moments earlier.

Take a moment now to think of a fear you have. See this fear in its fullness in your mind. Then become curious. Unpack this fear and search for its origins. Try to remember how long you've had this feeling. Was this someone else's fear, and at some point, you chose to adopt it yourself? Is there a part of you that believes that you would be incapable of navigating life if your fear became a reality? Challenge this perception. Would you really let this happen? Recall other times when you displayed your resiliency and inner strength, when you overcame something similar to what you are afraid of. Search for evidence of your power. It is there.

Check In with Your Breath

Something very interesting happens when we are struck by fear. We often think of fear as an emotion, but it is a physical reaction as well. This is what the fight, flight, or freeze response refers to. When a frightening or stressful experience occurs, the adrenal glands, which are located on top of both kidneys, produce adrenaline and cortisol hormones. The release of these hormones creates a series of physical responses, which include:

- increased heart rate,
- faster breathing or shortness of breath,
- butterflies or digestive changes,
- sweating and chills, and
- trembling muscles.

Of all these physical responses, the breath is the doorway into understanding what's happening in the moment. We can also shift our physical response to fear by using the breath, and if we can calm our physical response, then the emotions usually calm as well. We can always tell a great deal about how we're feeling by paying attention to our breathing.

Whenever you notice that your breathing is short and choppy, you're probably experiencing a stress response. But if you deliberately calm your breath, you can release that stress. Try it now. Recall a fear and let yourself really experience it in your body. Now begin to breathe with awareness. Place your hands on your belly and breathe deeply and slowly, inhaling through the nose and exhaling through your mouth. Breathe this way ten times, and then notice how you feel. Breathing in this way helps to relax the body, soothe the emotions, and calm the mind. This puts you in a better position to react appropriately in the moment.

Share Your Fears with Another

Within my first week of recovery, someone told me that a problem shared is a problem halved. Keeping your concerns and fears to yourself won't serve you in the end. The act of saying out loud to another human being exactly what you are worried about has the power to dismantle that all-consuming emotion. It takes courage to say to someone else, "I am afraid of ..." But the act of doing it will shift your perspective. Sometimes, even a tiny shift is enough to lighten our load and ease the burden of carrying our fears alone. We receive a gift by being heard, but we also give a gift when we share a deep part of ourselves with another.

Identify one or two people you trust; make sure to choose someone you know has your best interests at heart. Make a plan to share with them one or more of the fears you have. Ask them if you can call, write, or meet and have an honest talk. Trust in the knowledge that this special person or persons won't judge you for expressing your vulnerabilities.

• Deep-Diving Discovery Questions •

Self-inquiry supports us as we find greater freedom from fear, worry, anxiety, and shame. Shining a spotlight on the dark emotions we often hide robs them of their power. As you write your answers to these questions, be as honest as you can, and seek the insights that lead to solutions.

1. What are you most afraid of in your life? Be gentle with yourself as you look at this, as facing your fears is a courageous thing to do.
2. Are any of those fears based on past events? Take a moment to write down what comes to you when you consider this.
3. Ask yourself if any of your fears are based on circumstances or events that haven't been a part of your actual life experience, but that you anticipate might happen.
4. Who can you trust to share your fears with? Describe why you trust this person or persons.
5. What soothing practices can you use to help calm yourself when fears arise?

• Mindful Movement Moment: •
Spreading the Feathers

Before reading further, take a few minutes to recall the thoughts and emotions that discussing fear has raised, and then perform the mindful movement "Spreading the Feathers." It is important to take time right now to move your body. Through movement practice, you embark on a somatic journey of healing.

The purpose of this exercise is to release tension in the neck, shoulders, forearms, and hands, all places where stress manifests physically in the body. As you repeat this exercise, draw your attention back to the present, where great potential for growth and peace and courage resides.

In addition, with this and all the qigong exercises, if you feel inspired to repeat the movements longer than specified, please do. Repetition can induce a more meditative state.

1. Start by standing with your legs about shoulder-width apart.

2. As you ground yourself in this position, envision waves of calm gently washing over you.

3. Soften your knees, lengthen your spine, and lift the crown of the head toward the sky. As you do this, allow your arms to be along the sides of your body with the elbows and wrists slightly bent, fingers spread, and palms facing the ground.

4. Slowly draw the head to the left, bringing your ear closer to your shoulder (Fig. 3.1).

5. Slowly circle the head by bringing the chin toward the chest (Fig. 3.2).

6. Continue to slowly draw the right ear toward the right shoulder (Fig. 3.3).

7. Then slowly draw the head slightly back and up and over to the left again (Fig. 3.4).

8. Take deep breaths in through the nose and out through the mouth.

9. Perform this exercise at least three times to the right and at least three times to the left.

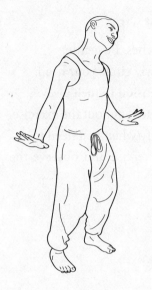

FIGURE 3.1

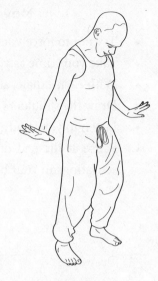

FIGURE 3.2

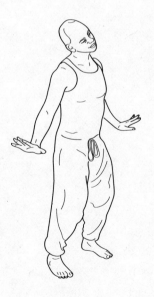

FIGURE 3.3

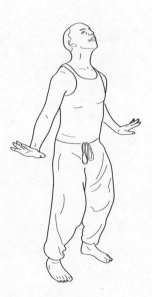

FIGURE 3.4

• Movement Tips •

- Try not to force your stretches. Be gentle.
- Take your time as you slowly circle your head.
- With each exhale, allow tension to melt away.
- Draw the shoulders down throughout the exercise.
- Listen to your body. Modify when you need to.
- Pause at the end of the exercise and observe the sensations in your body.

CHAPTER 4

• • • • • • • • • • •

MOVING PAST SHAME

If we can share our story with someone who responds
with empathy and understanding, shame can't survive.

— BRENÉ BROWN

I n this chapter, we are going to engage with the topic of shame because, frankly, it is the linchpin in the addiction journey. Shame is a painful emotion caused by consciousness of guilt, shortcoming, or impropriety. It is that little, dishonest voice inside that tells us that we are not good enough, that there is something inherently wrong with us and it is beyond repair. Shame touches the lives of everyone on the planet. This complex emotion does not discriminate. Shame is a part of humanity that few feel comfortable talking about. The process of understanding it and developing tools to deconstruct it and move past it are vital in our recovery journey.

Public shaming has a long history. It's been used in almost

every culture around the world to control or punish unwanted, unacceptable, or forbidden behavior. Among ancestral peoples, tribes would use abandonment and public shaming to punish members who left, strayed away from, or otherwise betrayed the perceived safety of the group. This same behavior is found in religious groups as well as most families. Search your own family history. Has the use of shame ever been used as a tool to control someone's behavior? In families, shame can be passed down through generations. In every family there are rules, many unspoken. We sometimes don't learn of the guidelines until we've broken them.

My recovery friend Keith is in his sixties and works as an interventionist. He helps people in the throes of addiction get the help that they need. He also counsels the families. He has long-term sobriety, and relapse is a part of his story. When I asked him about his early experiences navigating shame, he said:

> Shame was manufactured by the way that I thought about myself. When I was in first grade, I can remember coming home at the end of the day and staying awake all night because I was so terrified that my teacher didn't like me. That obsession that she liked everyone else and for some reason she didn't like me was developed internally. Shame was about the way I felt about myself. It had nothing to do with that first-grade teacher.

For most people, shame passes with time, just like other emotions. Feelings come and they go, like ocean waves along a beach. However, for addicts, alcoholics, and even codependents, shame tends to hang around indefinitely — most of the time without our awareness of its toxic presence in our life. This can lead to more difficult feelings and dangerous behavior. It can seem quite logical to walk along the path to self-destruction and addiction when we lack sufficient self-worth, feel ashamed of who we are, and don't believe that we matter or that we are worthy of love, respect, success, or joy. From this low point in life, self-medicating can seem like the only answer.

Keith shared how he dealt with shame for most of his adult life. "I went to any length to not feel shame. Regardless of what it took. Regardless of what I had to give up — important work meetings, things for my kids. All that stuff. I was self-medicating shame."

Much like Keith, I medicated my shame for years. It fueled my addictions, and it was unrelenting. For so long I felt very uncomfortable in my own skin. I didn't value myself and couldn't always see the positive things I brought to the world. I had tunnel vision and focused on what I perceived to be my flaws. Deep down I believed I was not worthy of love or good opportunities in life. There truly was a tiny voice whispering to me that I was not good enough to take up the space that I occupied on this planet. So, by the time I experienced my first night of drinking alcohol in a small pub in Germany, I was ready for relief. The intoxication I felt at age fifteen was a soothing balm for my wounded soul. From that night onward, I decided to pursue that feeling repeatedly, well into my early thirties.

For many people, self-medicating works for a long time, until it doesn't anymore. Eventually, a person realizes that they cannot fully escape their feelings, no matter how much they drink, how many drugs they take, or how much food they eat. The shame is always lurking just beneath the surface, waiting for an opportunity to pull them down like an undertow and carry them away to further depths of despair. Eventually, hopefully, people become clear that something needs to change, and it must start with their addictive behavior. Only once that is addressed can people effectively cope with the underlying shame. That was true for me. At first, I tried to address my mental health issues with one-on-one therapy, while at the same time refusing to change my addictive behaviors, and therefore my life didn't change much. It was during this time that I discovered how detrimental shame and other intense emotions are to the physical body, since they contribute to the following illnesses:

- addiction
- depression
- anxiety
- eating disorders
- compulsive behaviors
- perfectionism
- chronic pain
- digestive issues
- social phobias

Here is what Keith said about how his sobriety impacted his relationship with shame:

My relationship to shame began to shift because I repeatedly tried to figure out how I could get clean and sober. For me, that included going into one treatment center after another. I really believed that until I got to someone who dealt directly with the source of the shame, which was the anxiety, which was the OCD, which was all the other undiagnosed mental health issues that I had, I could not move past it. I got sober late in life, and I brought with me a huge bag of shame. Over the years and through several inventories and a lot of work, I'm not towing garbage bags filled with shame behind me anymore. They don't have control over me today at all.

Recovery Toolbox

Imagine for a moment a life where shame doesn't have a tight hold on you. Imagine yourself with the capacity to process it and move forward without it rattling your foundation in a significant way. It is possible, and by applying the suggestions below, you can make tremendous progress in moving past shame. This process belongs to you, and I encourage you to move within it at your own pace.

Own Your Story

Have you ever wished that your story was different or that certain life events hadn't happened? If you have, you are not the first and you won't be the last. We all have a story, a narrative of our lives. There will naturally be parts of it that feel more comfortable to remember, revisit, and recount than others. Some memories may elicit warmth while others might cause a queasy feeling in your gut or fill you with sadness. This is part of the human experience that we all share. Sometimes it can be challenging to accept this.

In 12-step recovery, much is said about acceptance. In the book *Alcoholics Anonymous*, it states the following:

> And acceptance is the answer to all of my problems today. When I am disturbed, it is because I find some person, place, or thing unacceptable to me, and I can find no serenity until I accept that person, place, thing, or situation as being exactly the way that it is supposed to be at this moment.

It has taken time for me to understand on a deeper level what acceptance means within this context. At first, I had the impression that acceptance meant that I had to like or agree with everything that happened or was happening in my life. That is not what acceptance means in the 12 steps or in recovery. The underlying message is this: Life holds many moments that can inspire difficult emotions like guilt, shame, anger, resentment, and disappointment, and we don't exactly get to choose how those moments will unfold or when. However, we can choose how we respond to life by owning our story and not running away from it or wishing that we had the life narrative of someone else.

I invite you to pause right now and reflect upon one event in your life when you felt shame. How do you tell that story? If you wish, take fifteen minutes or so right now and write this story down. Explore what caused you to feel shame. Be gentle with yourself as you reflect on this. Know that any shame you feel is only a small part of who you are as a person. We are all more than our shame.

Identify the Symptoms

According to sociologist Brené Brown, shame has physical symptoms. These might include our mouth getting dry, time seeming to slow down, our heart racing, twitching, looking down, and tunnel vision. These symptoms are different from one person to the next. So, if you learn your physical symptoms, you can recognize shame as it happens and get back on your feet faster. Take a few minutes to write down answers to the following prompts.

> I physically feel shame as [name sensations or parts of your body]...
> My shame symptoms include...
> When I'm experiencing shame, other emotions that arise are...
> If I could taste shame, it would taste like...
> If I could smell shame, it would smell like...
> If I could touch shame, it would feel like...

Then, in the moment, whenever you realize you're experiencing shame — stop. Take ten slow, deep belly breaths and repeat the following words to yourself: "I clear and release all my conscious or unconscious thoughts and feelings of shame." Afterward, notice how you feel. Notice if any energy has shifted for you.

Share Your Shame

According to Brené Brown, shame needs three things to survive: silence, secrecy, and judgment. As I say, shame hides in dark places, and the antidote is light. Sharing feelings of shame with others is how we shed light on those dark places and see what is there. Rather than making us feel worse, this is how we learn, accept, move on, and make better choices.

Here is an example from my life. It wasn't easy for me to enter graduate school to study traditional Chinese medicine. For one thing, I had a lot of alcohol- and drug-related damage from my past that I had to clean up to even be considered by the school. And I did that, and I worked hard to become a licensed acupuncturist...only to find out that that's not what I wanted to do after all. I had told everyone that "this is my future," and I had given up my whole life in New York to pursue this path, and I was terrified to have to admit, to myself and others, that I'd made a big mistake. I was filled with so much fear, embarrassment, and shame. I honestly didn't know if I was going to be able to stay sober through it. It was common for me to have panic attacks, and sleeping through the night was difficult.

During this remarkable and challenging time, one of the things that helped me greatly was sharing my shame with a few trusted people — close friends I felt comfortable enough with to admit my discomfort to. I was afraid to acknowledge my shame, but as soon as I did, I began to feel better. I felt like I could see things more clearly and I was able to breathe again, as if I had been literally holding my breath because of fear and shame. In part because of my willingness to speak up and not keep my shame a secret, I was able to let go of any judgments I had about myself and identify what I wanted to do next, and life improved.

Right now, I invite you to pause and identify one to three people you feel you can trust to share your shame with, people who would lend a compassionate ear. These could be friends, family members, or professionals, such as a counselor, teacher, or priest. If no one comes to mind, or no one who feels appropriate for what you have to share, consider finding a therapist (see "Seek Counseling" below) or call one of the many mental health hotlines that exist (see Resources for suggestions). They are staffed with trained professionals who are available to listen anytime you need to be heard. Consider which option may be right for you, then reach out and connect with those people. Decide the best way for you to convey this tender part of yourself to another person and follow through. Trust that the healing you need and deserve from this process is yours to have.

Laugh at Yourself

This type of healing around shame is serious work, but it's also possible to take it too seriously and to lose our sense of humor and wonder. Maintaining a sense of humor about life and its many ups and downs, and about ourselves and our many foibles, is also healing and can go a long way. Laughing at our problems, in addition to trying to fix them, is another way to express faith and confidence in ourselves that we will survive, come what may. Life contains a multitude of diverse moments, both highs and lows, so embrace them all, the same way we admire all the colors of a rainbow, which would be incomplete without any one of them. Take as many opportunities as you can to laugh. Laughter and smiling release endorphins, the same feel-good hormones that are released through self-massage, which is another reason laughter helps us relax and feel better. Make space in your life to laugh as much as possible.

Seek Counseling

Being in recovery requires courage, humility, patience, re-sources, and sustained effort. For many people, one important resource is seeking professional counseling. There are many good reasons to pursue therapy; understanding and releasing shame is just one.

One of many things that Keith and I have in common is the fact that we both sought counseling to address the underlying issues that fueled our addictions. I've heard it said in 12-step meetings that alcoholism is "cunning, baffling, and powerful," and I tend to agree. So is shame, fear, isolation, and all the other feelings and problems that lead someone to drink. Shame is insidious and will fester until it is addressed. However, when someone has lived with it for a long time, they don't always realize how it touches every aspect of life. Working with a well-trained therapist who is skilled at guiding people through re-covery is vital to effectively understand and deconstruct the causes of addiction and negative behavior for you.

Going to therapy is a big step. Seeking counseling is the act of asking for help, which is not an easy task. It is an acknowl-edgment that there is a problem and that we don't have all the answers. It is okay to not have all the answers. Thank goodness we don't have the responsibility of knowing everything. That would be exhausting, and it is impossible.

Finding a therapist that you feel comfortable and safe with is important. It's also important for you to set the pace of your therapeutic journey. Unpacking the origins of shame or any powerful emotion, understanding how it affects you, and de-veloping internal mechanisms to disarm it can't be rushed. The painful feelings we carry weren't created overnight, and they won't disappear in a day. It takes time and effort. Give yourself that time and space. I urge you to be brave enough to do this important, life-changing work.

If this is something that you are open to, set some time aside to research therapists who can help you address your needs. Ask trusted friends, family members, colleagues, or recovery professionals for referrals. That is a good place to start. Allow your inner wisdom to guide you on this part of your path. Self-compassion and freedom are waiting whenever we decide to take this step. The transformation we seek requires daily attention and help from a range of people.

Keith offered some final advice about coping with shame:

> My recommendation would always be, for dealing with shame, you have to identify the source individually. You may need professional help to do that. Then combine it with prayer, meditation, yoga, or any other mindful movement practice, as well as breathing exercises. Whatever it is that you may want to bring into your life to get you to a level that you want to start your day at. Those are the things I do to keep my shame in remission.

• Deep-Diving Discovery Questions •

I encourage you to dive deeper into how shame has affected your life. This self-inquiry will help you find greater freedom from shame and perhaps help you create more self-compassion.

1. Describe a few instances in which you felt shame. Then describe what you did with the shame each time. Do you observe any patterns?

2. In your family, has public shame ever been used as a tool to control someone's behavior? If so, describe how, and reflect on any ways this might have influenced the development of negative or addictive behavior.

3. Think about the times you have witnessed others express feelings of shame. Can you recall what it felt like to observe those moments and what emotions surfaced for you? Write down what you remember.

4. Staring into shame and learning to let it go is an important process. How can you celebrate yourself and the courage it has taken to do this work?

• Mindful Movement Moment: Shaking •

Before reading further, bring all that has been discussed and felt within this chapter to this mindful movement moment. Shame can take root in the mind, body, and spirit. We can encourage letting go of shame by doing the simple qigong exercise called "Shaking." This exercise can activate the energy within your body and release tension that you're holding. As you repeat this exercise, it will both energize and create a deep presence within you.

1. Start by standing with your legs about shoulder-width apart.

2. As you ground yourself in this position, envision waves of calm gently washing over you.

3. Soften your knees, lengthen your spine, and lift the crown of your head to the sky. As you do this, relax

your shoulders and allow the arms to be long at the sides of your body.

4. Begin to gently shake your hands, wrists, elbows, and shoulders.

5. Gently begin to pulse into your knees and feet. Allow the entire body to shake with a downward accent of the movement (Fig. 4.1).

6. Breathe in deeply through the nose and exhale fully through the mouth with an audible sigh.

7. Continue this shaking for the length of ten deep breaths. After the tenth breath, slow the movement steadily until you are eventually still. Close your eyes and observe the sensations within your body. You may feel a buzzing or tingling sensation. Be a witness to whatever you feel.

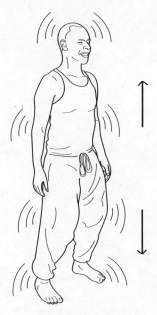

FIGURE 4.1

• Movement Tips •

- Keep your feet flat on the floor throughout the exercise.
- Allow the arms to remain long by the sides of the body and resist the temptation to shorten them as you shake.
- Focus on releasing tension with each shake and breath.
- Envision tension melting away in your neck, shoulders, upper back, lower back, and hips.
- Allow your breaths to be deep and slow. Try to make your exhale twice as long as your inhale.
- Listen to your body. Modify when you need to.

CHAPTER 5

. . . .

TRIGGERS & COPING STRATEGIES

Courage isn't having the strength to go on.
It is going on when you don't have strength.

— NAPOLEON BONAPARTE

Without a doubt, taking steps to change our life takes courage. In some ways, it can seem easier not to change and to go on doing the same destructive things we're accustomed to. At least these are familiar, and there is perceived safety in what is known. Stepping into the unknown and beyond the constraints we have created for ourselves is no small feat, but it is a worthwhile effort.

Once we have made the decision to change and started our recovery journey, we still may be tempted to fall back into old habits and patterns. Feelings, interactions, and events that tempt us are called *triggers*. A trigger can be anything; it is whatever makes us want to act out our addiction or engage in familiar negative behavior. It is fair to say that along a recovery journey, a person will be triggered many, many times and often in unexpected ways. For instance, we may be watching a film, and an actor drinks a martini in a way that makes alcohol look fun, glamorous, sexy, or calming, and suddenly we feel a craving to drink. We remember how it once soothed us, and even though we don't need soothing in that moment, we want it. Or at a family function, we get into a familiar disagreement with a relative who gets under our skin, and the interaction creates unrest within. We stalk off into the kitchen and are suddenly surrounded by temptation. We have had our disordered eating under control, but in that moment, we know that if we put even one chip in our mouth, we won't be able to stop. We are upset, and we know eating will soothe those feelings like nothing else. How do we maintain self-discipline? People who live with addiction can be caught off guard by cravings inspired by a person, place, or thing at any time.

Triggers Can Lead to Relapse

There is good reason why people with addictions can easily be triggered to relapse into addiction again. It all starts with the brain. According to the American Society of Addiction Medicine, addiction is a primary, chronic disease of the brain's reward and motivation circuitry. The brain regulates temperature, emotions, decision-making, breathing, and coordination. It also impacts physical sensations, cravings, compulsions, and habits. When chemicals like stimulants (caffeine, cocaine, nicotine), opioids (heroin, oxycodone), and sedatives (alcohol, diazepam, benzodiazepine) enter the body, they influence the brain. They cause people to lose control of their impulses or to crave the substance. The reward system of the brain is activated. In response to this brain activity, people continually return to the substance in order to unlock a wealth of euphoria. This leads to unhealthy behaviors and addiction.

The science of addiction to substances relates to all other addictions, including food, sex, gambling, and others. Researchers have found that the brain has the same chemical response to substance abuse as it does to compulsive, non-substance-related behaviors. In other words, people who get "high" from disordered eating, gambling, pornography, and so on, have the same chemical reaction in the brain as folks who drink and do drugs compulsively.

Thus, anyone in recovery for any reason is susceptible to the triggers that can lead to relapse. Indeed, relapse is a part of recovery for many. No one is perfect. We set good intentions to change, but we are only human, and we sometimes fall. When we do, it is important to get back up and carry on. Feeling triggered is very common in recovery, especially early in the process.

Knowing this, learn to recognize your common triggers, make a plan for dealing with them, and avoid them as much as possible (see the "Recovery Toolbox" below). In early recovery, I realized certain people triggered me to want to drink and do drugs. This was logical, since substances were the common thread that had run through those relationships. As a result, I decided I had to put distance between myself and those particular people. I had to choose. It was either my sobriety or those relationships. I chose my sobriety.

Ending a relationship is not always a choice a person

can make. It is not always a choice someone wants to make. We can't easily disconnect from every person and place that might be a trigger during our recovery. We may have spouses, children, and other relatives who are, in one way or another, closely tied to our addictions, and we may feel triggered whenever we are around them. Our job may be closely linked to our addiction or a source of triggers. These are all very complicated relationships and situations to navigate. Avoiding triggers is not the only criterion for deciding what to do when it comes to our family, our friends, our work, and where we live. In fact, it is not always advisable to make big changes like changing jobs, moving, or ending a primary relationship in early recovery. Doing so can add stress to an already stressful situation.

Stress itself can cause us to feel triggered, and being triggered can lead to panic or worry. However, while we can't avoid triggers, we can choose how to respond to them. Despite what our body and mind might be telling us in the moment, panic and worry are optional. We don't have to treat being triggered as a cause for despair. Sometimes we believe, to overcome strong feelings, we must respond to and resist them with equal strength, but that is false. Sometimes the best solution is to do the opposite: to allow the triggered feelings and do nothing. To remain calm, remember that this is all part of the territory, and wait until the feelings pass. And they will pass.

I had a conversation with my recovery friend Suzy about triggers and coping strategies. Suzy is a vibrant woman in her late fifties who's been married to her husband for over seventeen years. Suzy and I met in a recovery meeting in Northern California many years ago and became fast friends.

She believes strongly in the temporary nature of emotions. "It's all temporary. Whatever feeling or emotion that I have will pass. It will come and it will go, and there are a lot of tools that will get me through it."

Suzy has an interesting recovery story because she is juggling multiple addictions. She entered 12-step recovery to stop drinking and using drugs. Shortly after, she discovered an addiction to food that needed to be addressed as well.

I didn't put two and two together until after I stopped drinking and drugging, and then I was left with me and all my own feelings and emotions. I dove into recovery. In 12-step recovery there are writings about substituting sugar for the craving of alcohol, and my first sponsor even encouraged it. I do not encourage that with people I help in recovery because, for those of us with disordered eating, it's not a good suggestion. It's not a safe action to take. You must be very careful. Yet in the recovery meetings, there is the coffee and the doughnuts and the sweets, and those can be triggers. They often are. It wasn't until I put down the drinking and the drugs that I realized, ah, there was still more to look at.

Recovery Toolbox

Coping successfully with triggers boils down to three main things: practicing healthy physical self-care, knowing yourself and your triggers, and proactively making plans for what to do when you are triggered.

Suzy offered this advice for coping with addiction triggers:

Community, the hardest thing in the beginning of any
recovery. It is important to find a community of people
who get it. That will support you on your good and bad
days. That is an integral part of strong recovery. And be
open to new experiences like qigong, massage, yoga, or
whatever Eastern or Western modality that works for
you. Get out of isolation and into the movement. Move
a muscle, change a thought. It will help you get unstuck
and away from where you are.

Eat, Drink, Rest, Exercise

Your ability to handle any challenges depends upon you being
at your best. That means making sure that you are taking good
care of yourself by eating well, staying hydrated, getting enough
rest, exercising, and practicing good hygiene. When any of those
aspects of self-care are lacking, you are more at risk of being
caught with your defenses down when triggered. In 12-step
recovery, there is a saying, "Don't let yourself get too hungry,
angry, lonely, or tired." This is encapsulated in the acronym
HALT. If you are hungry, be sure to eat. If you are angry, call a
friend or someone you trust and talk about your feelings; same
if you are lonely. Reach out to someone who has your back. If
you are tired, take a nap or at the very least close your eyes and
breathe deeply for a few minutes. Being mindful of where we
are with our self-care habits is crucial. It is extremely difficult to
safely navigate a triggering moment if we are depleted and not
running on all cylinders.

Know Your Triggers

No two people are the same. What triggers one person may not trigger another. Suzy mentioned that she gets triggered by the available sweets at recovery meetings. I, on the other hand, am not triggered by that. Everyone is different. Emotional and environmental triggers can also inspire the desire to act out. Take some time to make a list of your triggers. Some common triggers are walking or driving past a bar you used to frequent, listening to music that you played while using, being around someone who is drunk or high, a stressful day at work (or pay-day), a disagreement or argument with another person, a cele-bratory moment, or even moments of boredom.

Don't fool yourself by thinking that you don't have triggers or won't be triggered. They are a very real part of addiction and recovery. That is why you need to anticipate what triggers you. You will have a better chance of responding in a healthier way if you do.

Create a Trigger Plan

Give some thought to how you will handle your triggers when they pop up. Come up with a simple plan of action. For in-stance, if a certain bar or neighborhood makes you want to act out, plan to take an alternate route to get to your destination. That is exactly what I had to do in early recovery, and it helped me avoid some tricky moments.

If you are concerned about wily encounters with others that may be triggering, consider role playing with someone you trust or even by yourself in the mirror. Practice saying whatever you will need to say in order to avoid succumbing to the craving and relapsing. It is better to practice when you aren't in a crisis so that you are ready when the stakes are higher.

However, we can't always anticipate triggers, so the most important part of any plan is anticipating what you can do to stop yourself from following through no matter what the situation. One strategy is to immediately pause and consider the consequences.

I've heard it said that if you stay in a barbershop long enough, eventually you will get a haircut. If you have a drinking problem and pick up the first drink, imagine that you will probably drink several more and get drunk. If you are a food addict and you eat a slice of cake, imagine how easy it will be to eat the entire cake. If you are a compulsive gambler and you walk into a casino, imagine the usual result: gambling all your money away. Consider the further consequences of guilt, shame, and regret that will result if you act out with your addiction. Every action has a consequence, but in moments of temptation, we sometimes indulge in magical thinking and decide that this time it won't. Don't kid yourself. When triggered, pause, think of how this path has always ended, and do something else (in your plan). This can save you a lot of trouble and heartache.

•   Deep-Diving Discovery Questions   •

To explore this topic further and discover insights, I invite you to journal your answers to the following questions.

1. Having support when you feel triggered is a good defense against acting out with your addiction. What type of support do you have in your life

today, and where can you find any further support you need?

2. What positive activities could you engage in to distract yourself from your triggers? Brainstorm the types of situations when each activity might be the most effective in the moment.

3. Imagine being triggered and responding to it successfully to avoid relapse. Write that story. Start with a situation that you would normally find triggering, and imagine using the tools from the "Recovery Toolbox": practicing good self-care, knowing your triggers, working the trigger plan you created, employing one of your support systems, and engaging in distracting activities to avoid acting out. Take your time and be detailed. See the moment clearly in your mind and feel it in your heart. See yourself handling the moment in a new, empowered, and effective way.

4. When you're finished writing this story, write about how this exercise made you feel.

• Mindful Movement Moment: •
Buddha Holds Up the Earth

Before reading further, do this simple qigong exercise called "Buddha Holds Up the Earth." Before you start, take a few deep breaths and recall some of the thoughts and emotions that were stirred up by this chapter. Now, take that emotional energy and apply it to this flowing movement, which is meant to enhance the lungs and the large intestines and create a sense of calm. It also creates more space in your rib cage to accommodate deep breaths, which tend to become tight, short, and shallow when we get caught up in our thoughts and emotions during stressful, triggering moments. As you repeat this exercise, it will draw you back to the present, where great potential for growth and peace resides. Use this anytime you're feeling triggered and need calm courage to make healthy choices for yourself.

As I mention earlier, this and the next four qigong movements are known as the Five Element Flow. Done together, they are designed to bring harmony between the practitioner and nature. They encourage the smooth flow of energy through all the meridian pathways in the body and affect the organs, muscles, tendons, and bones in positive ways. If you wish to create a longer qigong routine as part of your self-care practice, these five make a good grouping to consider.

1. Start by standing with your legs about shoulder-width apart.

2. As you ground yourself in this position, breathe deeply and envision waves of calm gently washing over you.

3. Soften your knees, lengthen your spine, and lift the crown of the head toward the sky. As you do this, allow your arms to be down, hands just in front of the hips with palms facing upward, and allow the elbows to be slightly bent and rounded. Relax your shoulders (Fig. 5.1).

4. As you inhale, draw the arms up the front of the body (Fig. 5.2).

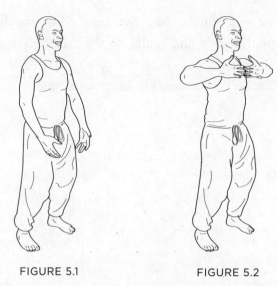

FIGURE 5.1   FIGURE 5.2

5. With the arms above the head, draw the shoulders down and keep a slight bend in the elbows while pressing the palms of the hands toward the sky. Slightly lift your gaze up to the hands (Fig. 5.3).

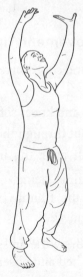

FIGURE 5.3

6. As you exhale, float the arms down the front of the body and return to the starting position (Figs. 5.4, 5.5).

7. Repeat this sequence at least twelve times.

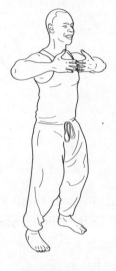 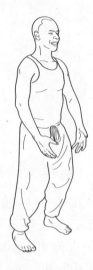

FIGURE 5.4   FIGURE 5.5

• Movement Tips •

- Take your time and coordinate the movement with the breath.
- Keep the elbows and knees soft the entire time.
- Breathe in and out through the nose, if possible.
- Pause the breath after the inhale and after the exhale.
- Reach through the thumbs when the arms are upward toward the sky.
- Notice any changes in your breath as you proceed.
- Pause when finished and observe the sensations in your body and your state of mind.

CHAPTER 6

. . . .

EXAMINING PERCEPTIONS

If the doors of perception were cleansed,
everything would appear to man as it is: infinite.

— WILLIAM BLAKE

In recovery, addiction is often referred to as a disease of perception. This refers to the unique way an addicted person thinks.
As Blake so famously noted, each of us perceives ourselves and
the world through our own limited individual lens, which affects the way we think and how we interpret what we see, hear,
touch, smell, and taste. After all, the only difference between an
optimist and a pessimist is what they make of an unfinished
glass of water: One person chooses to focus on abundance and
pronounces it half full; the other chooses to focus on lack and
says it's half empty. Two people, two perceptions, same object.

As a self-protective mechanism, the brain is hardwired
to focus on the negative. This applies to all people, but it is

particularly true for people who are challenged by addiction. Research has shown that those who become addicted generally have more negative perceptions about themselves, other people, and the world at large.

Negative self-perceptions often stem from low self-esteem. We frequently experience this as negative self-talk, or an inner monologue of self-defeating thoughts and ideas. Negative self-talk puts a stranglehold on a person and prevents them from believing in themselves and their abilities. These thoughts hurt and make recovery more difficult.

What Negative Self-Talk Sounds Like

During a conversation I had with my recovery friend Marti, we discussed perceptions, how tricky they can be, and the importance of examining them, especially in difficult situations. Marti is a married woman in her midfifties who lives in Colorado and works for an internet-based company. Her perspective on recovery comes from developing a debilitating codependent relationship with a recovering alcoholic and addict.

Here are some insights Marti shared:

Our perception of self affects everything. It shapes our entire world and how we see ourselves. So often when you have that negative self-perception, even though you may be projecting it onto other people, it really comes back to having to project that elsewhere because you were so uncomfortable with yourself. I think that often transcends addiction, but it certainly amplifies when someone is dealing with addiction. In my case, severe codependence. It must be my fault that my loved one has a problem, or it is because I wasn't strong enough, or I wasn't smart enough, or I made them angry. I did whatever. It was because of my perceptions of myself.

Marti's codependence arose in part from the false perception that she was powerful enough to control the uncontrollable — that is, the actions of another person. This reminds me of a suggestion that's often made in 12-step recovery: to get "right-sized." This means to learn that we are not the center of the universe. We are neither too big nor too small. We are encouraged to let go of any claim to greatness or grandiosity as well as to shame or unworthiness. To be right-sized, we place ourselves somewhere in the middle, worthy even while imperfect, strong even while vulnerable and limited.

According to the Mayo Clinic, negative self-talk comes in a few common forms:

- **Filtering:** We magnify the negative aspects of a situation and filter out all the positive ones. For instance, say it is Christmas and our partner gives us many gifts, all except for the one gift we were hoping for. All the gifts are lovely and thoughtful, which should make us happy. We have been showered with love and appreciation. Yet we focus on the one gift we didn't receive and feel disappointed and even critical of our partner for not getting it.

- **Personalizing:** When something bad occurs, we automatically blame ourselves. For example, say we made plans to go on a romantic date with someone, and they cancel at the last minute, citing a personal issue beyond their control. However, we assume they are lying to spare our feelings, since they obviously don't want to get involved with someone as unworthy as us.

- **Catastrophizing:** We automatically assume the worst. Say our application to attend a particular university is rejected. Instead of applying to other schools, we instantly assume we won't be accepted by any institution, that we'll never get the education and training we need to be successful, so we might as well give up on our dream career right now.

- **Polarizing:** We see things only as either good or bad. Nothing in between exists. A woman might feel as though she needs to be a size 6 to be desirable, and anything larger means she's unattractive. A man might feel he needs ripped muscles and six-pack abs to be attractive, and anything less makes him a loser.

Marti experienced lots of negative self-talk, which was predominantly about personalizing her loved one's addictions. Whenever her loved one chose to drink or use drugs, she believed it was her fault, even though she ultimately had nothing to do with their decision. This is what often happens in co-dependent relationships. A person's perceptions get so warped by negativity that it is hard to see the reality of a situation.

Changing Perceptions Is an Inside Job

Having negative perceptions can impact our physical and emotional health by creating additional stress. When all we do is focus on problems, and when we find problems in every situation, it drains our energy and keeps us from seeking solutions, even imperfect ones.

Some people believe that having a pessimistic attitude is simply being "realistic." They feel that life is challenging, disappointing, and unpleasant at times, and pretending otherwise is just a way to avoid "reality." The glass is, by objective measure, half empty.

However, that glass also contains water, and rejecting half a glass just because it isn't a full glass is self-defeating. It's like throwing all the water away without testing whether half a glass is all we need. Maybe half a glass is enough. In other words, changing our attitude and choosing to be optimistic isn't about pretending things are different than they are or good when they're not. It's choosing to be productive and make the best of what exists. This represents a far gentler, softer, and more humble way to navigate the ups and downs of life. All perception is limited, no matter what our attitude is, so the most practical, effective, and realistic approach is to always be open to the possibility that there is more beyond our small point of view. Things are almost always different, more complex, and less certain than we imagine. Believing our perceptions is like seeing the world through partially closed eyes at night; questioning our perceptions is like suddenly opening our eyes wide and viewing the world in the light of day.

Marti described how she became aware of her negative perceptions and began to make a change:

I just got to the point where I was so miserable with it all that something had to change. I couldn't go another day feeling that way. So, I had to begin looking inward because I had done everything I could to change everything on the exterior. How I acted, how I thought I could affect my loved one who was dealing with addiction. I changed all the behaviors I could possibly change and influenced them to the best of my ability, and we were both still miserable. So, what came to me was this must be an inside job because there is nowhere else to look. I then began a path of my own self-development. My own self-questioning, at least to look for relief. The big thing that shifted my perception regarding my addicted loved one was I couldn't understand the addiction because I wasn't an addict myself. Just coming to that understanding changed everything for me. That conclusion was life-giving.

Growth and change are an inside job. In order to change our circumstances and improve our lives, we have to first shift our negative perceptions of ourselves and the world. We have to go within and build a healthier emotional life.

Recovery Toolbox

Let's look at some ways you can challenge your beliefs and perceptions when they are interfering with living a fuller, more positive life. I recommend trying all these tools and gathering firsthand experience of their effectiveness.

Be Willing to See Things Differently

This tool is foundational for all the tools within this chapter, in this book, and on your recovery journey. In order to make any changes in our lives, we must be willing to try something new. Nothing changes if nothing changes. I encourage you to pause and make a commitment to yourself: to be willing to change any attitudes or perspectives that you discover are getting in the way of your happiness, your recovery, and your relationships with others.

Most people recognize willingness as necessary, but in practice, it can be surprisingly hard to embrace. Right now, I invite you to consider one situation in your life where there is tension or hard feelings. Do you recognize a sincere desire to have a different experience of that situation? Are you willing to see that situation differently? Sit with this for a few moments. Notice if any resistance arises. If so, be curious about it. Reflect upon its possible origins. In part, we can often disarm resistance simply by acknowledging it and by recognizing that willingness doesn't always occur instantly or overnight. This is a process. This exercise is about building awareness and preparing to change. Getting ready to get ready. Willingness opens the door to new possibilities.

Practice Appreciation and Compassion

To appreciate something is to recognize it with gratitude. This process of shifting perceptions requires that spirit of appreciation for your life and all the people you interact with. In a way, it is the essence of that shift: to switch from focusing on what we don't like to recognizing what, despite any flaws, is still good within us, in others, and in our situation. Doing this consistently takes practice, skill, and attention.

Right now, I invite you to think about a relationship or situation that is challenging you; it might be the same situation as above. In your mind, list two or three things that you can readily criticize, and then list two or three things about this person or situation that are favorable. Think of things you actually need or enjoy. To take an everyday example, I don't enjoy waiting in line at the grocery store. Who does? Is there anything to like about it? Well, when I consider it, I do enjoy the interactions I have with the cashiers, who are often kind, funny, and courteous people. I also enjoy and need what I buy. So instead of marinating in my aggravation at the inconvenience of lines, I can choose to focus on what I appreciate — the staff and the wonderful products — and change my entire experience.

Compassion is also essential to this process. As I say, embracing the challenge of shifting our beliefs and perceptions is no small task. Being willing to do this work requires courage and is to be commended. But of course, some days and some situations are easier than others. So practice compassion with yourself when you have moments of acting unconsciously and falling into old patterns, beliefs, and perceptions. They will pass and diminish with practice. I also invite you to extend compassion to all the people in your life as they struggle along their own paths. Not everyone embraces change and transformation, and those people may not like it when others change. We sometimes have people in our lives who want us to think, speak, and act in ways that are comfortable to them, that align with how they see us and the world. That's okay. But just because they aren't ready to embrace change doesn't mean we shouldn't.

Appreciation and compassion are essential tools for being able to shift your perspective in more productive ways. They can significantly transform your everyday experiences.

Whether big or small, each shift that occurs will empower you to move forward and grow in your recovery.

Move a Muscle, Change a Thought

A study conducted by scientists at the University of California at Berkeley concluded that humans have twenty-seven distinct emotions. That's far more than the six emotions that were once thought to be the extent of human emotional expression. But not all of these emotions are enjoyable, and some seem to grab hold of us and won't let go. Most of us are all too familiar with how heavy, negative emotions like anger, frustration, annoyance, irritability, fear, anxiety, and depression — in all their many shades — can get stuck inside. It is important to note that there are valid times to feel these things. In themselves, none are wrong. Every feeling we have is natural, but feelings are also meant to be temporary and to pass in time. Trouble arises when we won't let them go — when we get in the way of that process by ruminating, obsessing, and holding on to anger, grief, and so on.

Right now, I invite you to close your eyes and take five deep breaths. Breath in through your nose and out through your mouth. While breathing, check in with your emotional state. Notice where you are. Try not to judge what you are feeling. Just observe it. Whether you identify any lingering negative emotions or not, I invite you to turn on some of your favorite music and dance for at least two minutes. Dance, as the saying goes, as if no one is watching. Turn the speakers up as loud as you want, or put on your headphones, and enjoy your own personal dance party. While you dance, lift the corners of your mouth and gently smile. There are few things better in life than dancing and smiling. Afterward, pause and notice how you feel. Has your emotional state shifted? Do you feel elevated and energized in body and mind?

It is within your power to allow negative feelings to move through you and to transform them into positivity and peace, and it doesn't take long. Move a muscle, change a thought.

See the Good in Difficult People

We all have people in our lives we don't get along with easily. Some we can avoid, but others we can't, perhaps because we live in the same house with them or we work in the same office. Our difficult feelings are energy that can be felt, and this can cause the other person to respond in kind, which creates a situation that is tense, draining, and unsustainable.

In this moment, think about a person in your life who creates this challenging dynamic with you. Bring them to mind as clearly as possible. Allow your frustrations and your negative emotions and thoughts to surface. Then, put them aside and name at least one positive thing about the other person. No one is entirely bad or good. We all possess both positive and negative traits. Sincerely and compassionately, identify a genuinely positive trait, or several, that this difficult person possesses.

Then, the next time you think of or interact with this person, focus on that positive trait. In your mind, hold them up in the highest light you can in that moment. Release any resistance to doing this. This positive thought is also energy that can be felt, and before long, the quality of your interactions with this person will change for the better. They may begin to respond to you in a new way. Try this with all the relationships in your life.

Recognize Your Projections onto Others

Earlier in the chapter, Marti described how, when we have "negative self-perception," we can sometimes start "projecting it onto other people." Recognizing when we are doing this is an important part of changing our perceptions to foster awareness and a healthier approach to life.

A projection is when we criticize someone else for possessing a negative character trait that we refuse to acknowledge in ourselves. Of course, there can be multiple reasons why we dislike a certain person. We are not obligated to like everyone. But it's helpful for ourselves to recognize when someone we don't like or admire is actually mirroring a character flaw back to us that we won't admit we possess. The longer we stay in the dark about our shadows, the longer we can delay changing ourselves.

Right now, take a moment to think of someone you dislike. Bring them into your present-moment consciousness. Consider exactly what it is that you don't like about them. Now search within yourself. Do you recognize having those same character flaws? This can be difficult to acknowledge, but be honest. Have you ever done something similar in a different context, or felt the same impulse that seems so wrong, inexcusable, or abhorrent in the other person? I encourage you to do this exercise anytime you feel dislike or disdain for anyone in your life; search for ways these feelings might illuminate what lives in your own shadow. When you recognize a projection, extend compassion to yourself and the other person in that moment. The more we can do this type of inner work, the more we can change how we perceive ourselves and the world that we live in. We open to the truth and let go of false reality.

I asked Marti what advice she had for anyone who is struggling with negative perceptions. She said, "Give yourself a break. Society puts enough pressure on us without us doing that to ourselves. We are all perfect, divine beings regardless of the issues we carry around. Take time for you. Self-care must come first. Without it, we have nothing to share with others."

• Deep-Diving Discovery Questions •

Journaling is an excellent method for examining our perceptions to create a healthier recovery reality. Answer these questions with the goal to identify any limiting beliefs and perceptions that are undermining your recovery or hampering your joy.

1. Do you consider yourself an optimist or a pessimist? Describe why you view yourself in that way.
2. Where do you believe your view of yourself and the world comes from?
3. Have you ever felt like a victim of circumstance? If so, how have you been a victim?
4. When viewing that situation, or any difficult circumstance in your life, can you identify the role you may have played in creating that circumstance?
5. Examine one or two circumstances in your life and identify any examples of negative self-talk, then

consider how these situations might be improved by shifting negative perceptions.

• Mindful Movement Moment: The Fountain •

Before reading further, to integrate the teachings of this chapter into the body, mind, and spirit, take a few moments to do this simple qigong exercise called "The Fountain." Before starting, take a few deep breaths and recall some of the thoughts and emotions that this topic has stirred up, then take that emotional energy and apply it to this flowing movement.

The Fountain is meant to enhance the kidneys and urinary bladder and to facilitate more flexibility in the spine. It is designed to create a sense of relaxation in body and mind, allowing us to gently loosen our grip on any firmly held beliefs that can lead us to faulty perceptions. As you repeat this exercise, let it draw you back to the present, where great potential for growth and peace resides. Use this anytime you're feeling stuck in your beliefs and need to expand into a wider reality.

1. Start by standing with your legs about shoulder-width apart.
2. Soften your knees, lengthen your spine, and lift the crown of the head toward the sky. As you do this, allow your arms to be down at your sides. Relax your shoulders (Fig. 6.1).
3. As you ground yourself in this position, breathe deeply and envision waves of calm gently washing over you.
4. Gently shift your pelvis back and allow the arms to easily fall forward in front of the hips with the back

of the hands facing one another. The hands should
be about six inches apart (Fig. 6.2).

5. Tuck the tailbone under and shift the pelvis for-
    ward. As you inhale, slowly roll up through the
    spine while the hands and arms draw upward (el-
    bows pointing outward to the sides) in front of the
    torso. Relax the hands completely (Fig. 6.3). Once
    the bent arms are at the level of the shoulders, lift
    the head and stack it on top of the spine.

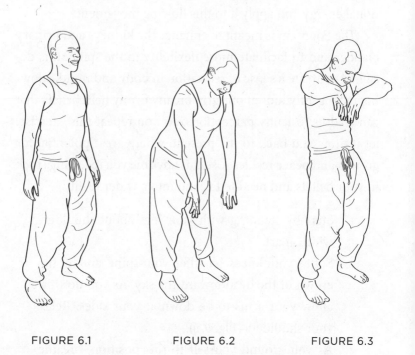

FIGURE 6.1   FIGURE 6.2   FIGURE 6.3

6. Lift the hands to the level of the head with the
    palms facing away and to the sides (Fig. 6.4).

7. As you exhale, open the arms out to the side, form-
    ing a T with palms facing downward (Fig. 6.5), and

slowly float the arms down to the sides of the body
and stand tall.

8.   Repeat the exercise at least twelve times.

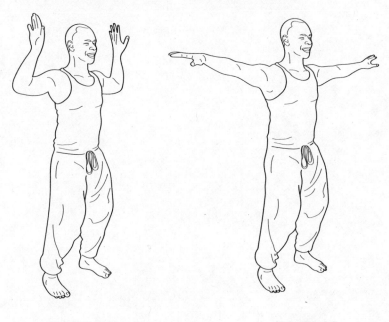

FIGURE 6.4   FIGURE 6.5

•   Movement Tips   •

- Coordinate your movement with your breath.
- Keep the knees softly bent throughout.
- As you roll up through the spine and lift the arms,
  be sure to relax the shoulders.
- Envision flowing water rising through the legs and
  spine and exiting out through the arms and hands.
- Envision the flow of the movement washing old
  beliefs away and creating space for new points of
  view to flourish.
- Allow your movements to be slow and fluid.

CHAPTER 7

. . . .

BUILDING SOCIAL SUPPORT

The wound is the place where the light enters you.

— RUMI

When I first conceived of this book, I knew that one of the most important things I wanted to highlight is the need for social support. Of course, it is a vital aspect of recovery, but it is also something that everyone needs all the time, and most of us aren't getting enough. For one thing, it reduces stress. According to a 2015 "Stress in America" survey conducted by the American Psychological Association, a significant percentage of people rate their stress level at 8 or higher on a scale of 1 to 10 (with 10 being maximum stress). Yet the survey found that those who had adequate social support rated their stress level at 5.

In the United States, independence and self-reliance are considered the ultimate virtues. Self-made millionaires are celebrated, and people are encouraged to "pull themselves up by their bootstraps," to go it alone and move forward under their own steam. Asking for help is often considered a sign of weakness.

Well, my experience is the opposite. A successful, rich, and healthy life always includes many people and resources. Asking for help is a sign of strength, and it's also smart. No individual succeeds without a community surrounding and supporting them.

Support Lifts You Up When You Are Down

For someone grappling with addiction, having a robust social support system can mean the difference between healthy recovery and relapse. People in early recovery can have difficulty coping with stress, which is why having a strong, supportive social network is so important. That network will look different for each of us, but in general it consists of some combination of family members, friends, peers, counselors, and other trusted people who can provide emotional support during times of hardship.

In early recovery I took a trip from New York to Boston to celebrate New Year's Eve with friends and old work colleagues. I was in recovery, my friends were not, and I understood that truth. At one point in the evening, I felt a wave of anxiety come over me when my friends opened a bottle of champagne. It wasn't shocking that they wanted to drink alcohol, but I thought I wouldn't be greatly affected by it. I was wrong. I suddenly had a strong desire to drink, and I feared I would relapse that night. I immediately called my friend Craig in New York,

who was sober; months earlier he had taken me to my first recovery meeting. Just hearing his voice over the phone calmed
me down as I anxiously stood outside my friend's apartment.
He assured me that just because I was feeling anxious and
triggered by the experience, I didn't have to drink over it. He
shared encouraging words as I took deep breaths. When we
said goodbye, I was then able to walk back into the party feeling confident and grounded, which helped me to enjoy the fes-
tive occasion. Having strong social support held me up when I
felt like I could not stand on my own.

My recovery friend Iliana is a married mother of three and
an animal lover. She has over a decade of sobriety. We had a
lively conversation about social support. I asked her about the
shift from being in active addiction to entering recovery and
the quality of her relationships at the time. Here is what she
shared:

> For me, I had to pretty much eliminate everyone from
> my life that I hung out with. Not one of those people
> had my best interest at heart. It was always about what
> I could get from them or what I could do for them.
> There was always some kind of motive behind it. I was
> in complete denial about my addiction, and my family
> eventually held an intervention for me. Thankfully, I
> was able to surrender at that moment, and it felt like a
> huge weight was lifted off my shoulders. That is really
> where my support started: having the support of my
> family to say, "It is okay and we know you need help;
> let us help you."

Iliana was very fortunate to have a supportive family that was willing to stick by her. Unfortunately, others have strained familial relationships that may have been countlessly tested by their addiction. For these people, it may require time and willingness to bridge the divide. It is hard work, but it can be done. It is not always easy to ask for help when we need it most. Sometimes we may feel driven to act as if we have everything under control while we are crumbling from the inside out. Perhaps it's the pressure to pull ourselves up by our bootstraps, as if that were possible. If you are a recovering addict, you know how difficult it is to bear the weight of this burden alone. What keeps many of us from reaching out is fear. Fear of judgment, fear of rejection, fear of change, fear of people — the many faces of fear. It is of great importance that we push past fear, humble ourselves, and let someone hold space for us to get well.

Building a Support Network

Iliana described what her first year of recovery was like and how she began to build her social support network, brick by brick:

> In my first year of recovery I went to an outpatient program, and I opted to attend 12-step meetings as well. I got a sponsor, and I met a bunch of women. They were amazing people, and I got used to calling them. At first it was very challenging for me because I didn't know what to say. It was very awkward, and I would literally say, "Hey, I'm just calling you because they told me to do so, and I don't have anything to say." The beauty of it

was they truly helped me by carrying me through the conversation. I got into the habit of reaching out without realizing that I was preparing myself for moments when I would really need someone to talk to because the shit hit the fan. I was ready for those moments where I would be in so much pain that I wouldn't want to reach out, but I was already in the habit of doing so. I didn't have to think twice about it.

What Iliana is modeling here is how she, despite her fear and awkwardness, got into the habit of reaching out to people when times were good so that her support was robust enough to guide her through the rough patches. She also illustrates how little she initially knew about building a support network, but she eventually learned how to build bridges between herself and other people. That is the goal for all of the suggestions in this chapter's "Recovery Toolbox."

Recovery Toolbox

Here are some ways to create more community in your life to bolster your recovery.

Be Honest about Needing Help

As I've mentioned, it is often difficult to ask for help. Do you find this to be true for you? The fact that you're reading this book shows a willingness to try something new and to reach beyond yourself. Take a moment to review your current situation. Are you struggling to manage the stresses of life? If so, would having more supportive people and resources available to you make your life more manageable? Consider your answers to those two questions as you review the other tools offered here.

It is impossible to change something we won't admit exists. Therefore, be truthful and honest with yourself about your need for help. This is the first step to building a more supportive community and creating a more comfortable life.

Don't Let Fear Stop You

Take a moment to check in with yourself and inquire whether you are afraid to reach out for support. If so, what exactly is it about asking for help that scares you? Please be specific. The more you know and acknowledge, the better off you will be. Fear is a tricky emotion. It seems like it protects us, but it can also stop us from doing what is most helpful simply because it's unfamiliar or makes us feel vulnerable. Having support can help us navigate any difficult emotions that arise from day to day. Creating a life-affirming community can help take the edge off daily stresses and lighten our load.

Next, ask yourself what actions you are willing to take today to push past any fear to get the help you need. Here are a few suggestions:

- Make a list of who might help you. Only put people on this list who have your best interests at heart.
- Pick up the thousand-pound phone and call one or two of those people. Let them know what you are trying to do and invite them to help in any way they can.

- Call a recovery or support hotline to discover what resources are available to you (see Resources).

Determine What You Want and Need from Others

After spending time in active addiction, it can be challenging to trust our ability to determine what type of help we need from others in our recovery. We wasted precious time making choices that were not in our best interest and led us deeper into addiction. Today, I encourage you to trust your ability to make better choices. Your better judgment led you to this book and process. I invite you to pause right now and take a few deep breaths. In the silence, ask yourself what your top two needs or wants are from others. For instance, do you need someone who will be present for you without judgment? Do you need someone who will provide wise guidance without trying to control you, who will allow you the dignity of making your own decisions? Perhaps you need someone who will gently remind you when you begin to show signs of old, destructive behaviors. Support from others can provide healthy peer pressure. Friends can help us make better decisions for our recovery and overall well-being. Perhaps, especially initially as you rebuild, you need help with the practical things in life. Assistance with things that we generally take for granted, like transportation, grocery shopping, and cleaning our home, can feel like small miracles when we are lifting ourselves up from being down. Whatever your needs and desires when it comes to support, write them down to create more clarity for yourself. This will help you be specific and concrete as you ask others for what you need.

Attend Regular Recovery and Support Meetings

Did you know that there are at least thirty-eight different types of 12-step programs in existence around the world? All of them are modeled after the steps first created by Bill Wilson and Dr. Bob Smith in Akron, Ohio, in 1935. The magic of recovery meetings is that they gather together people from all walks of life around a common purpose: to help themselves and one another gain freedom from their addictions.

Since 1935, a lot has changed. Of course, 12-step programs don't suit everyone, and many other types of recovery groups have sprouted up. They include groups like Self-Management and Recovery Training (SMART), Women for Sobriety (WFS), Secular Organizations for Sobriety (SOS), LifeRing Secular Recovery, and Moderation Management (see Resources for contact information).

The point is, you don't have to create a support group for your recovery all on your own. A wide range of recovery and sobriety groups already exists, and all you have to do is show up (in person or online). These groups don't replace your existing supportive community of friends and family, but they can be a vital additional resource of caring people who know what you're going through because they are going through it themselves. I urge you to search for a group that will address your needs. Help is just a few steps, a phone call, or a click away.

Iliana shared with me how important the relationships she developed through meetings have been for her:

> In the fellowship I'm a part of, we have something called Bloodlines. They are sober families created through sponsor/sponsee relationships. We all come together

in very intimate settings where we speak freely about things we wouldn't necessarily share at meetings. We meet once per month, and we rotate whose home we will meet at. We come together, eat, talk, and listen to one another. It is such a wonderful foundation that I formed in the beginning of my recovery. I came to trust those women and I could share anything with them. They helped me through one of my most difficult times in sobriety.

Follow Your Interests and Passions

There is more to life than addiction and recovery, so pursue your interests, hobbies, and passions, especially any that you dropped or lost once addiction took over. Choose those things and activities that bring you joy, and look for ways to join existing groups or communities. Recovery support groups, activity clubs, sports teams, and classes are great ways to foster healing, supportive connections with others around shared interests.

Take a moment to consider the healthy interests you enjoy, or always wanted to try, and write them down. Maybe that includes sports, bike riding, hiking, music, dancing, art, or knitting. Then consider joining a club, enrolling in a class, or volunteering for a local charity or organization that could use your able hands and talents. Doing any activity of your choosing creates pleasant experiences with others and builds healthy relationships over time.

That said, people in recovery often feel socially awkward, since their addiction has isolated them, and if you feel that way, know that you are not alone. In the past, I have felt that way as well. Alcohol and drugs were a social lubricant for me, and in sobriety I had to learn how to connect with others without them. One tool that has helped me over the years is to connect with others by being curious about their lives. Ask open-ended questions related to the activity:

- How long have you been participating in this?
- How often do you do it?
- What do you enjoy most about it?

Often, participating in the activity itself is enough to break the ice. In this way, we can create healthy relationships with others who have no connection to our addiction or recovery.

Be Patient

It takes time to build strong social support. Give it time and do not give up. Especially when you feel like doing so. If you practice patience with yourself and others as well as keep an open mind and heart, you will be amazed by the remarkable community you will build. A community that will stand with you during the highs and lows and everything in between.

Iliana offered this advice about trying to build a new support system:

My suggestion would be to find the fellowship that best suits you. I would suggest making ninety meetings in ninety days. To sit at the front of the room and no matter how embarrassed you are, raise your hand and introduce yourself. Because within those ninety days, you will see a lot of the same people. You will hear their stories. You'll get to see what these people are about, and you can be the judge of who you feel most comfortable with. By raising your hand and saying that "it is very hard for me to reach out and I need help," you will be surprised how many people will be there willing to help. They will send you texts in the morning, call you and pick up your calls, and carry that conversation, like they did for me in the beginning. So again, for me it is about creating a whole new support system and brand-new people in my life. I was able to meet those women I mentioned earlier, who are still in my life today. I met my sponsor through making meetings on a regular basis. One meeting every day for ninety days. That would be my suggestion.

• Deep-Diving Discovery Questions •

A supportive community doesn't appear by magic or happen by chance. We have to identify what we want, who we want, and then cultivate those relationships. These self-inquiry questions are meant to help you do that. Insights and solutions await on the other side of this journaling exercise.

1. Consider one or two people you trust, who have your best interests at heart, and write about why they make you feel safe and at ease. What do they do to make you feel loved, appreciated, and supported?

2. Consider the possibility of attending a recovery

meeting or support group. What would you want out of it? What type of group would make you most comfortable? If you have any reservations about them, describe the cause of your resistance.

3. Looking ahead or at the big picture, what would your ideal social support network look like? What is currently missing in your life right now, and how might you start to create it?

• Mindful Movement Moment: •
Tree Sways in the Wind

Before reading further, please do this simple qigong exercise called "Tree Sways in the Wind." Take a few deep breaths, recall some of the thoughts and emotions that were stirred up by this chapter, and then begin. This flowing movement is meant to enhance the liver and gallbladder and is designed to help alleviate daily stress. It also creates strength and flexibility in the body and mind. Life is filled with unexpected events, and in order to endure these changes, we must be resilient. Use this anytime you're feeling stressed and need to ground yourself like a tall tree with deep roots in the earth.

1. Start by standing with your legs about shoulder-width apart.

2. As you ground yourself in this position, breathe deeply and envision waves of calm gently washing over you.

3. Feel the feet firmly rooted into the ground like a tree. Soften your knees, lengthen your spine, and lift the crown of the head toward the sky like the

branches of a tree. As you do this, allow your arms to be down, hands just in front of the hips with palms facing upward, and allow the elbows to be slightly bent and rounded. Relax your shoulders (Fig. 7.1).

4. Turn from the hips and waist to the right and carry the shape of the arms with you.

5. As you inhale, float the arms up the right side of the body with your palms facing upward (Fig. 7.2).

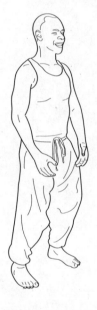

FIGURE 7.1

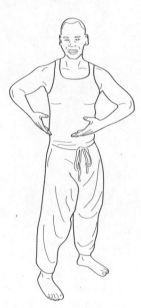

FIGURE 7.2

6. Hover the fingertips of both hands an inch above the crown of your head, with the backs of the fingers facing one another, and point the bent elbows out to the sides. Maintain the arm position as you now face forward, standing like a tall tree in full bloom (Fig. 7.3).

7. As you exhale, lift the arms and hands up and away
    from the head and then allow them to float out-
    ward and down with the palms of your hands fac-
    ing away from you (Fig. 7.4) until the arms are low
    and resting in the starting position.

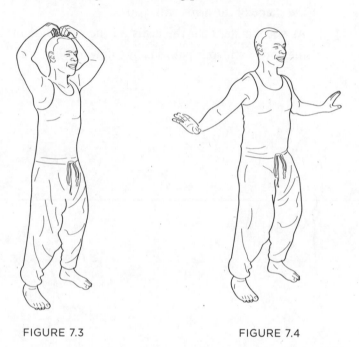

FIGURE 7.3   FIGURE 7.4

8. Repeat the movement to the other side. Then re-
    peat the entire exercise at least twelve times.

• Movement Tips •

- Take your time and coordinate the movement with
  the breath.
- Keep the elbows and knees soft the entire time.

- Breathe in and out through the nose, if possible.
- Relax the shoulders down as you lift the arms.
- Soften the hands and be mindful of excess tension you may be holding.
- Notice any changes in how you breathe as you progress through the exercise.

CHAPTER 8

. . . .

LIVING IN GRATITUDE

Acknowledging the good that you already have in your life
is the foundation for all abundance.

— ECKHART TOLLE

Choosing gratitude can have an enormous impact on our lives. When we focus most of our thoughts and energy on what we consider to be wrong, we miss the fertile opportunity to recognize what favorable things are simultaneously blessing us. This process of recognition sets in motion a new awareness and appreciation for the people, places, and things in our lives that make it rich and fulfilling. This is part of what it means to change our perceptions and the way we view life, as discussed in chapter 6. Optimism and gratitude go hand in hand, as do pessimism and ingratitude.

An author and professor of psychology at the University of California at Davis, Robert Emmons has done extensive research on gratitude. He states, "The practice of gratitude can have dramatic and lasting effects in a person's life." Emmons has found that practicing gratitude has positive effects on our body, mind, and social connections; it improves our health and well-being in numerous measurable and immeasurable ways. Some benefits are stronger immune systems, lower blood pressure, more feelings of joy, and a greater sense of social connection, among many others. We have nothing to lose and much to gain by turning our attention to the positive aspects of life.

However, despite decades of research into the positive effects of gratitude, some people remain skeptical. Some say that gratitude leads to complacency or is just a naïve form of positive thinking. Some believe that expressing gratitude isn't appropriate — or even possible — when we're in the midst of suffering, or that we must be religious to be grateful. I once shared some of these myths and misconceptions about gratitude. However, I eventually became willing to put aside my skepticism and explore this practice, and I encourage you to do the same. The willingness to embrace gratitude can lead to an abundant life.

The Fertile Ground of Gratitude

I know from experience that when we're in the midst of addiction, we focus primarily on the misery in our lives, and those discontents fuel the addiction. When our energy focuses exclusively on the problem, we create more of the problem. However, when we allow the sunlight of gratitude to shine its rays into the dark corners of our life, we can uncover solutions, see the good things that exist, and create fertile ground for more of it to grow.

In the 1990s, I was watching an episode of the *Oprah*

Winfrey Show in which Oprah spoke passionately about the practice of keeping a gratitude journal. I had never considered such a thing. She said, "I know for sure that appreciating whatever shows up for you in your life changes your personal vibration. You radiate and generate more goodness for yourself when you're aware of all you have and not focusing on your have-nots." I was moved by this and attempted to start a gratitude practice while in the throes of my addictions, but I was not successful. It was like taking a daily vitamin pill to be healthy while still poisoning myself with alcohol, drugs, and a steady diet of negativity. It just doesn't work. Once I got sober, a recovery buddy suggested that I consider approaching life with an attitude of gratitude, and so I began again.

My recovery friend Kristen is a sober, single mother and business leader. Since meeting her many years ago, I've marveled at her positivity and the way she is able to find the good in life. She explained that she also had to be encouraged to change a negative mindset:

> When we first get into recovery, it is hard to be grateful because of the destruction we've inflicted upon ourselves. It is easy to focus on the negative. But when I had someone teach me and require me to send a gratitude list daily, my mind began to shift a lot. My experience also began to shift.

The Distance between Us and Gratitude

For people at the beginning or in the middle of a recovery journey, pivoting toward gratitude can feel like a push. I, too,

doubted whether gratitude would change my life in a meaningful way. Yes, I saw the practice working for others, but I
saw myself as "terminally unique," meaning that I had a belief
that the situations I was facing were somehow different from
those of everyone else. Therefore I had a right to wallow in my
discontent.

Kristen described one possible source of resistance: "Some
people are opposed to practicing gratitude. Many people are
invested in the state that they are in because it is familiar and
comfortable to some degree. Life consists of change, which is
disturbing for us all. It is nice to know what is going to happen,
but unfortunately that is not life."

Self-centered fear makes it hard to be grateful. Often, our
fear isn't about anything that is actually happening, but we fear
things that might happen in the future. Gratitude brings us
into the present and asks us to focus on what we are grateful for
in this moment. Like many people, Kristen had to experience
this for herself to understand how transformative it can be.

I was going through a difficult time. I had a lot on my
plate in the beginning, and when I thought about it, I
would spiral downward. So, my sponsor had me send
her a list of five things I was grateful for upon awak-
ening. First thing in the morning. Initially, I doubted
it would help me. I decided to do it to appease her. I
really didn't think it was going to have any effect on
me whatsoever. And I found it was like a magic bullet
because I really tried to make my list different every
day and detailed. Regularly identifying things to be
grateful for is such a simple exercise, but it takes time
to build the habit. I started expressing gratitude for the

basics and it grew from there. I would have to sit there in the morning and think of things deeply. What was I grateful for? Was someone in my life a cause for me to be grateful? Was there something about the weather? Was something like an act of kindness or something that happened to me a cause for gratitude? Sometimes I had to be grateful for the strength to be able to write a gratitude list at all.

When we earnestly engage in this process, it begins to re-wire the brain. Scientists have discovered that whenever we express or receive gratitude, our brain releases dopamine and serotonin, two neurotransmitters that are some of the so-called feel-good hormones because they make us feel better. By practicing gratitude every day, we can help strengthen these neural pathways and create positive changes within ourselves.

Kristen now touts the benefits of practicing gratitude to anyone who will listen:

Being grateful is the most important thing I do in a day. I think out of all the tools I've ever used for myself, this has been the most effective because it changes my mood, my outlook, and gratitude begets gratitude. If you start feeling gratitude, suddenly it seems like you have more to be grateful for.

Despite her initial reservations about the effectiveness of a gratitude practice, Kristen pushed forward and gave it a try. At first, her efforts were small, and some days she could only get herself to be grateful for the weather or for the willingness and strength to be grateful at all. That was enough to set things in motion. Keep that in mind for yourself as you explore the tools I offer next for developing an ongoing gratitude practice in your everyday life.

Recovery Toolbox

The first two recovery tools are complementary exercises. They build a deep and personal sense of gratitude within, and in time, this overall feeling will infuse every part of your life and recovery. The last two exercises are also complementary: They prompt you to share those feelings with others. By bringing gratitude along with you as you do the work of recovering yourself, it softens the rough edges of any challenge and deepens your appreciation of every win.

Take a Gratitude Break

As an experiment, take a gratitude break right now. Think of five things you are grateful for today, and write them down. Then take a few moments to reread what you've written and consider why you are grateful for these things. That's all, but give yourself an extra moment to take in the quiet power of the exercise.

Next, try this prescription: Continue taking a gratitude break once a day for the next week. This is a great way to start your day, but there is no wrong way or bad time to do this. You can be grateful for anything, from the tiniest, most mundane things to the largest, most precious things. As you continue through each day, take moments to reflect on the list, and if you feel inspired, add to it. You can never be too grateful.

At the end of the week, compare how you feel about the practice now to how you felt initially. Has anything changed? Give this practice time to alter your perspective until seeing the world and your life through the eyes of gratitude feels natural all the time.

Take a Photo

This fun exercise is an alternative type of gratitude break. As the saying goes, sometimes a picture is worth a thousand words, so instead of (or in addition to) writing down what you're grateful for, take photos throughout the day on your cell phone camera of people, places, and things that inspire gratitude in the moment. Make it a fun game for yourself. Hunt for things that inspire gratitude. Capture images that are meaningful to you. If you find yourself having a fun and enjoyable moment, take a photo of that moment — of yourself, another person, or the place you are.

Like the previous exercise, try this for a week, and at the end of each day, take a few moments to review that day's gratitude pictures. As you do, recall the positive feelings, joy, and inspiration that caused you to take each photo. Cultivate those feelings of gratitude in your awareness, and see if they carry over into the next day. Notice if your perspective on gratitude changes, and modify these exercises in whatever way inspires you the most.

I often take photos of the sky, plants, flowers, my cats, or food that I am cooking. Taking the photos always fills me up with awe, wonder, magic, and joy, and I tap into those same feelings when I revisit the photos. I remember how grateful I am for so much in my life. Every time you look at your photos, they will surely do the same for you.

Share Your Gratitude

The next two exercises are ways to extend the spirit of gratitude you are cultivating by sharing it with others. This will enable it to grow. Each day, after you have created your gratitude list, or as you review your gratitude photos, share some or all of these moments and thoughts with someone in your life who would appreciate the practice. Let inspiration guide you to share expressions of gratitude with whoever is appropriate, but I also recommend developing a consistent exchange of gratitude with one or more persons. It's fast and easy to do this by calling, texting, or emailing, and it's a wonderful practice to do early in the day because it sets a joyful tone for the hours that follow.

If you have already created a gratitude list in "Take a Gratitude Break" above, I invite you to share one or more of those thoughts with someone today. Consider who might be a good choice to join you in a daily practice of gratitude for one week and ask them. Then, at the end of the week, check in with yourself and the other person. How do you both feel? Has sharing gratitude improved your experience or affected your connection? Depending on how you feel, you can decide whether to continue the practice of sharing gratitude.

For two years, I shared my gratitude lists with friends both inside and outside of recovery. It started off as an exchange between myself and a couple of people, and it grew to be a group of seven with whom I shared my daily list. Some participated for a long time, and others were a part of the journey briefly.

Some sent their lists back to me, while others gratefully received my lists but never kept one for themselves.

As Robert Emmons has found, gratitude improves interpersonal relationships in all areas of life. Expressing gratitude creates positive emotions, primarily happiness. What a transformative experience it is to share happiness with others. It is an energy that uplifts all who are touched by it. In time, everyone gets caught in a "gratitude flow" where the energy of thankfulness moves effortlessly through you and everyone around you.

Write a Gratitude Letter

Lastly, consider writing a letter of gratitude to someone who is important to you and share with them how much you appreciate and value their presence in your life. This is meant to be a deeper, more profound expression of gratitude, so take time to consider who to write to and what to say. That said, the note does not have to be long. Simply explain the intention behind your correspondence and share one or two things about the person that you are grateful for and why they are so meaningful to you.

Of course, it's natural to do this with people we love and feel comfortable with. But this can also be a powerful exercise to do with someone important with whom we have a less-comfortable relationship. They may be surprised by your outreach, and most people enjoy pleasant surprises. That said, if writing a letter to anyone is a stretch for you, consider writing the note today and waiting to send it at some later date. This task alone will fill you with a new sense of thankfulness that can inspire profound change.

•   **Deep-Diving Discovery Questions**   •

To explore this topic further and discover insights, I invite you to journal your answers to the following questions.

1. Do you have any resistance to the idea of a gratitude practice, or of expressing gratitude to others? Explore the source of any ambivalence, anxieties, and fears you might have.

2. Describe times when you've found it easy to express gratitude, and describe times when it has been hard.

3. After writing a list of five daily things to be grateful for, take extra time to explore what about them makes you grateful. Be specific and personal and see if there is more to discover.

4. Do the same thing with your gratitude photos. At the end of one day, write about how they make you feel. Explore and express your feelings, and be as descriptive as possible.

5. What surprises, if any, has this practice of gratitude revealed to you?

•   **Mindful Movement Moment: Cloudy Hands**   •

Before reading further, I encourage you to take a few deep breaths, recall some of the thoughts and emotions that arose while reading this chapter, and do the qigong movement called "Cloudy Hands." This flowing movement is meant to enhance the heart and small intestines and to help balance the emotions. It also creates flexibility and strength in the hips and spine and encourages a release of tension in the forearms and hands. Life presents challenges that test our ability to keep our hearts open and live with a sense of joy and compassion. Use this anytime you're feeling unable to see your circumstances through the lens of gratitude.

1. Start by standing with your legs about shoulder-width apart with soft knees.

2. Lift both arms to shoulder height in front of you. Round the elbows as if you are wrapping your arms around a tree. Allow any tension in the hands to melt. Hold your arms gently as if they are clouds floating in the sky. Lengthen the spine as the tailbone drops and the crown of the head lifts. Soften the shoulders down away from the ears. As you ground yourself in this position, breathe deeply and envision your heart and mind rising above any worries of the day (Fig. 8.1).

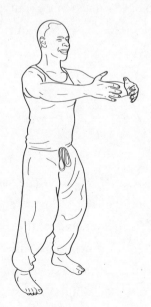

FIGURE 8.1

3. As you inhale, shift the body weight to the left as you turn from the hips and waist to the left. Allow the right arm to lower in front of the hips while the left arm remains at shoulder height (Fig. 8.2).

4. As you exhale, shift the body weight to the right as you turn from the hips and waist to the right. The right arm will lift as the left arm lowers (Fig. 8.3).

5. Repeat twelve sets of this exercise, swaying to both the right and the left over and over. When finished, relax the arms down, pause, and notice what you feel.

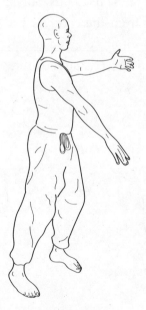
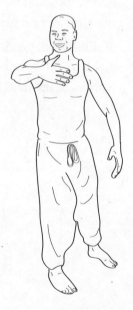

FIGURE 8.2   FIGURE 8.3

• **Movement Tips** •

- Take your time and coordinate the movement with the breath.
- Keep the knees soft throughout.
- Soften the hands and be mindful of excess tension you may be holding.
- Remember to maintain the space between your arms and body as you wrap your arms around the imaginary tree.
- Turn the body from the center.

CHAPTER 9

• • • • • • • • • • •

FINDING FAITH

Faith is taking the first step
even when you don't see the whole staircase.

— MARTIN LUTHER KING JR.

When I began my recovery journey, it started by taking one step. I didn't know exactly what would follow and yet something propelled me forward, urging me to trust the signs and signals that I had been heading in the wrong direction. This took faith because, indeed, I couldn't see the whole staircase. I just knew I had to keep walking and trust that there would be ground beneath my feet. This was not always easy, but it was possible because I knew my old way of living wasn't serving my highest good. My intuition whispered to the deepest part of me that I had to step into a different future that held the potential to heal my body, mind, and spirit. Of course, I had no idea where to begin, but I called my friend Craig, who was and is a beautiful model of sobriety, and he took me to my first recovery meeting. I was anxious and afraid, but my gut told me to follow his lead and trust the process I was entering. I had an elementary understanding that I had made it this far and there must be a reason for it. I didn't have to know why, but I did have to stretch myself to be okay with not knowing.

Initially, embracing a spiritual or religious faith wasn't on my radar. Yet I quickly realized that trusting in a power greater than myself was going to be an important asset in my recovery. This became even clearer when I began reaching out and receiving more support from others in recovery. Nearly everyone relied on some type of spiritual faith, though how they expressed their faith differed. In one form or another, it was a strong belief in a benevolent, loving power greater than ourselves that cares for and guides humanity and all life. Personally, the God that I was brought up to believe in didn't suit me as an adult trying to learn to love myself and get sober. I had to dig deep and decide what was and was not true for me. Everyone I knew was doing the same — they were adopting the faith that resonated with them. Ultimately, the decision to believe or not believe belonged to me, just as it belongs to you. In this chapter, my intention is to encourage you to cultivate faith in whatever terms are meaningful to you, but without trying to persuade you to accept my or anyone else's particular beliefs.

For many people in recovery, a spiritual faith contributes to positive outcomes. Studies show that people with a religious or spiritual faith of some kind have higher optimism about life and resilience to stress. Faith in a caring presence, power, or spirit outside of oneself can also help people feel less alone and less lonely. All of this is important for people in recovery. Sometimes the only thing that stands between us and the substance or behavior we are addicted to is our faith and the strength we garner from it.

While I feel it's important to rely upon faith in a Higher Power to guide us when direction is needed and to comfort us when life becomes hard to endure, there is another form of faith that is also necessary: trust in oneself.

Trusting Yourself

In early recovery and beyond, it can be challenging to trust ourselves because of the countless broken promises we have made. When we look in the rearview mirror, we may see a trail of incidents where we broke our word to ourselves and to others. This can be discouraging, but it is possible to overcome that feeling and learn to trust oneself again.

In an enlightening conversation I had with my recovery friend Jennifer, we discussed finding faith in recovery. We talked about the challenges, opportunities, and solutions on the road to trust and faith. Jennifer is in her thirties and works as a wellness professional, and she struggled with trust early on.

Well, I think something that addicts share between each other is that we didn't really trust ourselves for as long as we could remember. So, trusting a recovery process or a family member, a friend, or someone like that is sort of a foreign concept because we have not trusted ourselves in so long. To ask us to trust something outside of ourselves is even more impossible. Trust is a word we didn't understand in our addiction, and it is going to take almost just as long as when we were addicted to something to trust something to heal us.

I learned a transformational lesson about self-trust within my first year of sobriety. I was offered an opportunity to join a theatrical touring company. At the time, I was just getting comfortable with my new life. My cravings to use alcohol and drugs were getting under control, I had a supportive community around me, and I enjoyed a solid routine of recovery meetings. I had found my sober groove, and the thought of leaving the safety and security of that was scary to me. I didn't trust myself to be out on the road alone and maintain my sobriety. I searched my soul for answers, talked it over with my sponsor, and I decided to turn down the offer. I wasn't ready. This felt like the right thing for me to do.

However, I kept open the possibility of taking such a bold step in the future. Three months later, another offer appeared, and I felt ready to accept. Creating trust within oneself happens in stages, just as Jennifer described. Bit by bit we gain more confidence in knowing what the next right action is to take. During the time I spent on the road I proved to myself that I was trustworthy and could keep my commitment to stay sober no matter where I was or what I was doing.

Spiritual Faith

What helped me while traveling with the touring company was my faith in a Higher Power. I think of this power as an energy that is a part of everything on this planet and within the universe. I see this energy as a force that loves me and wants me to experience my highest good. Whenever I felt uneasy, fearful, or stressed while away from home, I turned to my Higher Power. Experience had already taught me that I could trust myself to not fall back into my addictive behavior, even when tempted or challenged, but I still needed more support at times.

After about six months on the road, I received some disturbing news. Someone from my addictive past, whom I had not seen in well over a year, was joining the touring company. This sent shock waves through me. Memories of drunken and drug-filled days and nights filled my mind. It was difficult to escape them. I felt a twisting sensation in my gut when I thought of the hurt, pain, and destruction that took place between myself and this person. From the moment that I heard of their impending arrival, my appetite diminished, and I couldn't sleep through the night. I felt guilt, shame, remorse, and anger over the thoughts, words, and actions from my destructive past. Hurt people often hurt people. After days of this distress, I sought counsel from trusted friends, and I also turned to my Higher Power to seek some intuitive guidance and relief from my anguished state. What this led to was a newfound confidence that all would be well. I strengthened my faith on a deep level that no matter what happened, I would be okay, and I would be able to maintain my sobriety during that challenge. I also had a new understanding of the word *control* and how it weaves in and out of my life.

In active addiction I responded to things that I had no control over by using substances to affect how I felt. I could change how I reacted to the world by anesthetizing my body and mind. I did the same thing when the irritant originated within me. Drinking alcohol and using drugs gave relief during times when I was fixated on a difficult emotion. Through chemical reactions in my body, I tried to take control of myself in all ways. In recovery, I still wrestle with the idea or illusion of control, but without chemicals. I now recognize that feeling in control helps me feel safe. In sobriety, I consistently and carefully determine what I have control over and what is beyond my influence. I find healthier ways to feel safe and self-soothe. Today, what I have dominion over is myself, my attitude, and my perceptions. This I know for sure; it is my mantra. Everything else is out of my reach. Having trust and faith in myself and a Higher Power helps me loosen my controlling grip when I feel uneasy about the unpredictability of living in the world.

Before I found recovery, I felt the presence of that Higher Power in my life, even while I suffered through active addiction. However, I did not always trust it. My quest to stay sober made me willing to trust it more. I believe it was waiting for me to love myself as much as it already loved me.

Jennifer had a similar experience with her Higher Power:

I believed in a power greater than myself prior to recovery, so I think I am a bit unique. I fall into the category of recovering addicts who did. I, for as long as I can remember, did believe in an energy and a power much greater than myself. I always knew that there was an energy out there. Not necessarily controlling everything but guiding and watching over. I call that energy God. I know that there is something greater than myself at work. Mostly because I didn't die several times in my addiction. Something was taking care of me. Something continues to care for me and keep me sober.

Jennifer refers to herself as "unique" because she entered recovery with a certain amount of faith. Not everyone has that. Faith is a complicated subject for many people. Some people have a difficult history with God and religion, and those experiences can make the process of finding faith challenging. It can make a person hesitant to move forward into treatment and recovery. But spiritual faith doesn't have to be based on any form of established religion. The universe or nature itself are both powers that are greater than humanity, greater than any individual. Life itself is mysterious and awe-inspiring, and some people feel most comfortable focusing their reverence on this force. All that matters is that someone develops an understanding and a faith that reflects what holds meaning for them. Faith is always personal. Developing trust and faith is itself a process that requires faith and patience.

Patience is an attribute that still does not always come easy for me. The process of finding faith takes time. The hours between day and night can't be rushed, and neither can this. Falling into the mire of addiction doesn't happen in the blink of an eye, and neither does building a strong recovery and faith. How long it takes to go from not trusting oneself to eventually creating a firm bedrock of self-assurance depends in part on the attention and effort paid to this shift. Along the way, moments of doubt and despair are inevitable. So much is learned during those uncomfortable times if we are willing to be students of life. Practice patience and keep your focus on the goal of creating a new relationship with yourself and with whatever you consider your Higher Power.

Jennifer shared more about her relationship with hers:

When I think about the relationship between me and my Higher Power, I think it is personal and private. Before I got sober, nothing was ever private in my life. I thought my using was private, I thought my relationship and my disasters were private, but I am certain that everyone could tell that I was not well, and I was hurting. Especially the more insightful and intuitive people. Having this private and personal relationship with something you can't see allows you to believe in something that is not material. Addicts carry a lot of stuff with them such as drugs, alcohol, and other destructive behaviors with the intention of getting high, and they hold power over us. We have a relationship with those things. So now if that relationship can be with a Higher Power, we just know that we are okay. We just believe that something larger than us exists, and we aren't in control of everything. We alleviate ourselves of that responsibility and we agree to step back. We aren't used to that.

Letting go of control, as Jennifer described, can be very difficult for people in recovery. As I did, many people use addiction as a way to control their bodies, their feelings, and their surroundings in order to feel safe. This sense of dominion might be an illusion, but while intoxicated, we can fool ourselves. However, we can ignore this fact and fool ourselves during recovery, too. We can get to a point of overcoming our addiction and feeling powerful and safe — that is, until some upsetting event beyond our control reminds us to have humility. Believing in a power greater than ourselves is this reminder that we don't call all the shots in life, that much is beyond our control. Thank goodness we don't have the responsibility of controlling everything that happens.

Allowing a Higher Power to have a positive influence in our life is not always a simple task. I asked Jennifer what she would recommend to anyone who is struggling to trust and have faith today. Here is what she shared:

> I've always said to people that were questioning whether they wanted to get sober or change their life or be in recovery, "Well, you've made it thus far. You're living and you're breathing now. So can you get behind the idea that it's going to work out because it has worked out thus far?" On a deeper level, I truly believe that there is no wound so deep that we can't heal from it. I tell people that faith is one of those things that you don't have to believe in because it just exists. And proof of that is you've made it this far. You have made it through your trials and tribulations up until a point where you are talking about it. I believe that you are spiritual because you are alive. So, to the people who are doubtful about faith, I say, "You don't have to believe. Faith already knows about you." People say they don't understand the "greater power than me" thing, and I say that is okay because this power knows about them. So, feel safe in this moment and decide later if you want to figure it out.

Recovery Toolbox

Try these tools and see if they help you find faith along your recovery journey.

Name Your Higher Power

I invite you to take this moment to name a Higher Power for yourself. If you already have a defined spiritual faith, that's wonderful. If you don't, that's also wonderful, but take this moment to consider what might qualify as a source of spiritual faith — a benevolent force greater than yourself. Perhaps, for you, it might be nature, the laws of science, love, the universe, music and art, or our collective humanity. Don't feel like you need to make a final decision right now, but choose some personally meaningful concept that holds mystery and power and affects all life in significant ways. Follow where your heart leads. In 12-step recovery rooms, people often refer to the group as their Higher Power. For them, they regard the word "GOD" as an acronym for "group of drunks." Finding comfort in the wisdom and power of a group that has their best interests at heart has helped countless people. Whatever you choose for now, know that your conception of a Higher Power will evolve over time. It will grow as you grow.

Once you've named a source of faith, reflect upon this Higher Power throughout the next few days. Consider the attributes of this faith that truly speak to you. Take time to do this chapter's "Deep-Diving Discovery Questions" and write about what you find. What qualities define this power for you, and when do you experience them? For instance, I consider my Higher Power to be loving, caring, wise, humorous, powerful, ironic, compassionate, mysterious, and much more. My faith helps to move me forward to become the best person I can be.

If this exercise is difficult, that is okay. This is where patience comes to play. Can you find the willingness to revisit this tool in the coming days or weeks? See if you feel a shift take place within you over time. Be open to discovery, and try to have faith even if you don't have faith. Remember what Jennifer said: It doesn't matter if you believe because faith already knows about you, and that sometimes is enough.

Breath Prayers to Build Faith and Trust

There is an ancient practice of linking our thoughts to our breath. Using the mind and body to build faith. Some refer to the practice as "prayers from the heart" because it frees the practitioner from formulating prayers and allows them to rest in the pureness of intention and the physiological act of breathing. This practice builds upon the simple breath practice I share in chapter 1 (see "Deep Belly Breathing," pages 27–28) and applies it to faith and trust. This practice is known to bring people closer to their Higher Power and create a feeling of calm and wellness.

One version of breath prayer is to call to mind a word or phrase that is meaningful to you in the moment. Then on both the inhale and the exhale, think of that word. Try to embody that word or phrase in your breathing. Another approach is, on the inhale, to think of a word that corresponds to something you need more of in your life, like love, peace, joy, or courage. Then, on the exhale, think of a word that corresponds to something you want to release from your body, heart, and mind, such as anger, resentment, fear, stress, or loneliness. Choose whatever words and phrases are meaningful to you. You can also say the word silently in your mind or chant or even sing the word as you breathe. Do whatever works best for you. Over time the prayer becomes a part of you on a deep level. It leads to the release of the emotional traps we fall into as humans and helps us walk toward an elevated state of being that embodies positivity and enlightenment.

Recently I found myself in a moment of worry and anxiety, and I practiced this form of breath prayer. My words were *peace* and *fear*. I inhaled to draw more peace into my life, and I exhaled fear to release that emotion. Eventually, as I repeatedly said those words in my mind in time with my deep, slow breaths, fear and worry slipped away, and I became filled with a sense of peace and trust that all was well.

Try this simple practice now and see where it leads you. If it helps, try this for a few minutes every day for a week and see how you feel. This is truly a remarkable practice.

Collect Things That Inspire and Encourage You

One way to build faith is to surround yourself with things that inspire and encourage you. I'm a firm believer that my Higher Power speaks to me through other people, things that I read, nature, music, and art. For instance, I might feel down and suddenly hear a piece of classical music that stirs my soul and renews me, allowing me to see my day in a whole new light. I receive inspiring recovery quotes via email every day, and some touch my heart deeply. They address something that has been weighing on me and provide me with insight and hope. Sometimes, that is all I need to help me walk down the mysterious staircase of recovery and life.

Today, start your own collection of inspiring things and adorn your home and work space with them, so you see them often. They can help lift you up and carry you forward like wind in your sails. Print or write down quotes that hold meaning for you. Put up pictures or photos or art, or surround yourself with plants and flowers. Create playlists of your favorite music or of music that you find uplifting. Every day, see, touch, and contemplate sources of inspiration.

Be creative and have fun. Invite faith and your Higher Power as an everyday presence through the things you bring into your life and surround yourself with. Do this every single day and begin now.

•   Deep-Diving Discovery Questions   •

As you respond to the following questions, be honest and curious about your answers. You may be surprised by what you discover.

1. Describe several times when you successfully trusted yourself. What about these situations led to this trust?
2. Describe several times when you felt doubt and did not trust yourself. What about these situations caused doubt?
3. What does spirituality mean to you?
4. Where does your spiritual power show up in your daily life?
5. How do you define wisdom? Where do you look for wisdom in your own life?
6. When have you felt most connected to your spiritual side?
7. What mantras or guiding principles do you, or might you, use in your spiritual life?

• Mindful Movement Moment: •
Pebble in the Pond

Before reading further, take a few deep breaths and recall some of the thoughts and emotions that have been stirred up by this chapter. Feel what comes up for you, and apply that emotional energy to this exercise, "Pebble in the Pond." This flowing movement enhances the stomach and spleen and is designed to help ground and center you. It also creates mobility in the hips, strengthens the legs, and helps improve digestion. Recovery comes with many twists and turns along the path. There will be many distractions and unexpected events that will try to discourage you. It is important to stay grounded, centered, and stable. This movement will help.

1. Start by standing with legs about shoulder-width apart and toes pointing forward.

2. Ground yourself into the moment by feeling your feet firmly planted on the floor. Soften your knees, anchor your tailbone toward the ground, lift the spine, and reach the crown of the head toward the sky. Relax the arms by the sides of the body with palms facing the outer thighs. Relax the shoulders and soften the elbows. Breathe into this powerful posture (Fig. 9.1).

3. As you inhale, bend the elbows and point them back and allow the palms of the hands to rise to the level of the hips, with the palms facing forward (Fig. 9.2).

4. As you exhale, slightly shift the hips back as the arms fall forward with the palms facing down in front of the hips. Reach the hands forward and

then out to the sides as if the hands were gliding on the surface of a pond and drawing a horizontal circle, creating ripples with your touch (Figs. 9.3, 9.4).

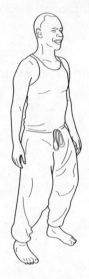

FIGURE 9.1

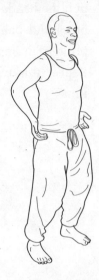

FIGURE 9.2

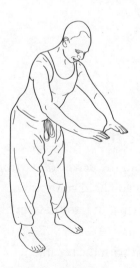

FIGURE 9.3

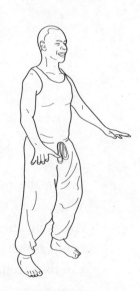

FIGURE 9.4

5. As you inhale, shift the hips forward to stack the hips directly over the feet, shoulders over the hips and head on top of the spine. At the same time, pull the hands back toward the hips with bent elbows and palms facing forward, re-creating the position in step 3 (Fig. 9.5).

6. Repeat this two-position sequence at least nine times.

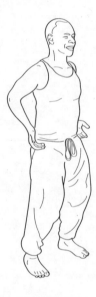

FIGURE 9.5

• Movement Tips •

- Initiate the movement from the pelvis. Move from your center. This is where you hold your power.
- Allow lightness in the arms and softness in the hands as they move.
- Coordinate the movement with the breath.
- Keep the knees soft the entire time.

EPILOGUE

Congratulations on reaching this point in your journey. I hope that this book has met you wherever you are on your road to wellness and provided a road map of inspiring stories, tools, and practices to help you recover the self you lost to addiction and to live a more conscious and joyous life. The time you have invested in this work is a small yet significant part of your total efforts to change your life. Everything that you have learned or gained from this experience is now a part of you, and nothing can change that. It is something that you can always revisit to help you go deeper into the many layers of recovering you.

When I began my recovery journey, I remember feeling so many emotions. I had a steady train of thoughts running through my mind, and many of them weren't productive. It was challenging to make peace with my mind and body in the absence of mood- and mind-altering substances. Prior to sobriety, I spent a lot of time and energy running a few steps ahead of uncomfortable thoughts and feelings. Somehow in those early days I managed to fall forward instead of backward and created a solid recovery foundation for myself.

One day, a trusted friend hugged me tightly and encouraged me to forgive myself for any harms I had done to myself while in active addiction. They urged me to keep on forgiving as I accumulated hours, days, weeks, months, and years of recovery because I would continue to occasionally have lapses in judgment and sometimes regret things I might say or do. At that time, I was holding on to so much judgment and resentment toward myself for treating my body poorly, for stuffing my feelings down so far that they became toxic in my system, and for not always honoring and respecting others along the way.

We're often taught to forgive others without much thought of granting that same mercy to ourselves. Please hear me now: Forgive yourself if any part of you still holds judgment and resentment toward yourself. I know this is not always easy to do, but it is worth trying your best to do so. Allow that to be the springboard to your brighter future. If you knew better or could have done better than you did, you would have done so. It is impossible to move through life perfectly without making "mistakes."

I believe that mistakes are not bad things. They are opportunities to grow, learn, change, and evolve, if we choose to do so. With that said, nothing is wasted, and nothing is truly lost. It is all meant to lead us to becoming more of who we *truly* are: the *self* without all the projections from the outside world or layers of protective armor that we developed because of the trauma we have endured in life. This armor makes it difficult to spread our wings and fly and find the freedom we seek.

My parting wish is that this work will give you a sense of freedom to approach your life in a new way. If you don't quite feel that sense of freedom right now, that is okay. *Recovering You* is here for you to tap into as much and as often as you need. When you feel inspired, circle back to the beginning or to any other part of the book and see if it leads to new insights and unlocks parts of you that you may not have been ready to release days, weeks, or months ago. The freedom you seek might be right around the corner or a little further down the road.

Never give up. Life is in session. It will occasionally throw unexpected things at you, but difficult circumstances will never be made better by acting out in self-destructive ways. They will only be made worse. Stay the course and ask for help when you need it. You may not be exactly where you want to be right now, but you are a few steps closer than you were before. That is progress, and striving for progress, not perfection, is what's productive and healing. This approach will serve you well while traveling along the beautiful and ever-changing road to wellness and recovery.

ACKNOWLEDGMENTS

A multitude of individuals were integral to the process of making of this book. Also, many have been key contributors to my life's journey and have helped shape the person I am today and prepared me for the monumental task of becoming a teacher, healer, and author. Thank you to each person on the list below, and I send deep gratitude and love to all others who have supported me and my work through the years.

First and foremost, I must acknowledge my Higher Power for guiding me from my first breath up to this moment. My faith has led me through the darkness and into the light, and I will be forever grateful for the presence of a power greater than myself.

Next, I thank my husband Lee Harris for his unyielding love of who I am and support for all I do in this world. From the day when I began to write short stories about my life and recovery, you have always been an enthusiastic cheerleader and audience. I would be remiss if I didn't also mention our cats Obi and Bebe, who have been by my side throughout my creative process, always providing fun and tender distractions exactly when I needed them.

Thank you to my sister Terri Alexander, who has always loved me for who I am and believed that I could do anything I set my sights on. Thank you to the maternal figures in my life, my mother Dottice Barnes and my mother-in-law Meryl Harris. Deepest appreciation for the interest you both have shown in my writing and the encouragement you showered upon me while I wrote this book.

To my deceased father James Washington, who loved me dearly and displayed pride in his eyes and voice whenever in my presence: You were one of my greatest teachers by showing me a valuable life lesson. We are only as sick as our secrets, and we heal by telling the truth. Witnessing your struggles helped me commit more deeply to my recovery.

My friends Douglas and Dianna generously provided a quiet Midwestern retreat for me to write, rest, and recharge in. The gifts of community, nature, and support were priceless.

Thank you to my dearest friend Natalie Rand. Your ability and willingness to listen to me as I navigated this momentous period of my life and career have meant so much to me.

Many thanks to my recovery friends who graciously shared their experience, strength, and hope in the pages of this book. The voices of Randee, Bill, Marti, Keith, Iliana, Suzy, Kristen, and Jennifer have helped create a supportive and nurturing community for me as well as the readers of this book. Thank you all for saying yes.

Without the help and guidance of my sober mentors, I wouldn't have the abundant life that I have today. Thank you, Craig L., Fabrice M., Bill T., Steve A., Bill R., and Barry K., for being powerful examples of how beautiful and complex a sober life can be and always delivering messages of hope.

My recovery was enhanced beyond measure by the time I spent with my sober fellows who allowed me to share what had been so freely given to me. Thank you, Jeffrey L., Brian L., Reagan C., Duane B., Skip J., and Nathan S., for being wonderful sober brothers and teachers along my recovery path.

Thomas Yogeshwar Leichardt was my initial qigong teacher. From my first day of study, I was guided to remember who I truly am through the energy medicine of qigong. Thank you, Thomas, for giving me a solid foundation. I later met other master teachers who taught in ways that spoke to me and allowed me to flourish and grow as a student and a teacher of this healing modality. Thank you, Lee Holden and Dr. Roger Jahnke, for all the ways you support my life and the lives of others through your work.

Many thanks to all the great teachers I had the pleasure to learn from while studying massage. Julie Porter, Jeff Rockwell, Curtis Hisao, and Conrad Santos shared their gifts and tools with me, and I now will pass them on to others through this book.

The opportunity to create this book wouldn't have been possible without a hunch that Georgia Hughes had about me and my ability to write. Thank you, Georgia, for reaching out and inviting me into this remarkable world of publishing. I am grateful to Jason Gardner, Tracy Cunningham, and the rest of the wonderful team at New World Library. I appreciate all that you've done to bring *Recovering You* to life.

Many thanks to my friend Tanya Malott, who photographed me for the book's cover. Thank you for sharing your artistic eye and skill with me and the world.

To my incredible writing coach and editor Jeff Campbell, thank you. I knew that you were the guy for me when I saw your name on a list of potential editors. My intuition led me to contact you, and I am so glad I did. You know how to celebrate the wins in the creative process as well as to hold space for the writer when we hit a rough patch. Your ability to pull out the best in a writer and get to the heart of a story or teaching is brilliant. I appreciate you and your immense talent.

Erin Posanti, thank you for your beautiful illustrations. It was an absolute pleasure to collaborate with you on this book. Your images have helped me bring this movement practice to countless people seeking its healing power.

Debra Evans, thank you for saying yes when I asked for your assistance with putting together a winning book proposal. I appreciate the time, energy, and love you gave to me and this project in its early stages.

And lastly, thank you to the amazing team at Lee Harris Energy and Steven Washington Experience — Noah Perabo, Marti Bradley, Wendi Cohen, Anna Harris, Chelsea Paiz, Adam Perabo, Rebecca Hall, Davor Bozic, Patrick Keily, Nick De La Cruz, Trent Barfield, and Meredith Perabo. By being masterful at what you all do, you allow me to focus on what I do best. I am grateful beyond measure.

RESONANCES

RESOURCES

Addiction Recovery Programs

12 Step–Based Programs

Al-Anon, https://al-anon.org
Alcoholics Anonymous, https://www.aa.org
Cocaine Anonymous, https://ca.org
Co-Dependents Anonymous, https://coda.org
Gamblers Anonymous,
    https://www.gamblersanonymous.org/ga
Narcotics Anonymous, https://na.org
Overeaters Anonymous, https://oa.org
Sex & Love Addicts Anonymous,
    https://www.slaafws.org

Non-12 Step–Based Programs

Buddhist Recovery Network,
  https://www.buddhistrecovery.org
LifeRing Secular Recovery, https://lifering.org
Moderation Management, https://moderation.org
Secular Organizations for Sobriety,
  https://www.sossobriety.org/#home1-section
SMART Recovery, https://www.smartrecovery.org
Women for Sobriety, https://womenforsobriety.org

Hotlines and Helpful Resources

National Institute on Drug Abuse (NIDA),
  https://nida.nih.gov
National Suicide Prevention Lifeline
  (800-273-8255), https://suicidepreventionlifeline.org
**Substance Abuse and Mental Health Services
  Administration** (SAMHSA),
  https://www.samhsa.gov

Books on Recovery, Addiction, and Qigong

Cohen, Kenneth. *The Way of Qigong: The Art and Science
  of Chinese Energy Healing.* New York: Ballantine Books,
  1997.

*The EZ Big Book of Alcoholics Anonymous: Same Message,
  Simple Language.* Gainesville, FL: BeaconStreetUSA,
  2015.

Gates, Rolf. *Daily Reflections on Addiction, Yoga, and Getting
  Well.* Carlsbad, CA: Hay House, 2018.

Griffin, Kevin. *One Breath, Twelve Steps: A Buddhist Path to Recovery from Addiction*. Sounds True, 2015, compact disc.

McKowen, Laura. *We Are the Luckiest: The Surprising Magic of a Sober Life*. Novato, CA: New World Library, 2020.

Rosen, Tommy. *Recovery 2.0: Move Beyond Addiction and Upgrade Your Life*. Carlsbad, CA: Hay House, 2014.

Shapiro, Rami. *Recovery — The Sacred Art: The Twelve Steps as Spiritual Practice*. Woodstock, VT: Skylight Paths Publishing, 2009.

Smith, Bob, and Bill Wilson. *The Big Book of Alcoholics Anonymous*. Augusta, KS: Lark Publishing, 2013.

ABOUT THE AUTHOR

S teven Washington is a qigong, Pilates, and meditation teacher, as well as a writer and speaker who lives a life of recovery and is passionate about helping others as they navigate their own recovery journeys. Washington performed on Broadway in Disney's *The Lion King*. His love of dance and movement led him to become a Pilates instructor and certified neuromuscular massage therapist, as well as a certified Lee Holden Qigong instructor. He teaches Core Qigong, a fusion of Pilates and qigong, online weekly through his website. He also teaches qigong internationally and has held more than fifty events around the world. He lives, teaches, and writes from the Los Angeles area.

www.stevenwashingtonexperience.com